NEUROSCIENCE RESEARCH PROGRESS

OLIGODENDROCYTES

BIOLOGY, FUNCTIONS AND ROLE IN THE PATHOLOGY OF DISEASES

NEUROSCIENCE RESEARCH PROGRESS

Additional books in this series can be found on Nova's website
under the Series tab.

Additional e-books in this series can be found on Nova's website
under the e-book tab.

NEUROSCIENCE RESEARCH PROGRESS

OLIGODENDROCYTES

BIOLOGY, FUNCTIONS AND ROLE IN THE PATHOLOGY OF DISEASES

DANA SWANSON
EDITOR

New York

Library of Congress Cataloging-in-Publication Data

ISBN: 978-1-63483-330-1
Library of Congress Control Number: 2015944489

Published by Nova Science Publishers, Inc. † New York

Contents

Preface

Oligodendrocytes have multiple functions in the central nervous system including mechanical support of neurons, production of myelin sheaths and uptake and inactivation of chemical neurotransmitters released by neurons. Consequently, oligodendrocytes could be involved in the pathology of a number of neurodegenerative diseases. The first chapter of this book examines the range of disorders in which oligodendrocytes play a significant role. In the second chapter, the authors review the effects of microglia on oligodendrocytes in both physiological and pathological conditions. The third chapter focuses on cell transplantation for myelination of axons in spinal cord repair. In the fourth chapter, the authors review data showing the induction of some plasticity of olidogdendrocytes (OL) by growth factors and axon proteins in vitro. Finally, the last chapter is an examination of the potential uses of anti-S100B therapies to treat myelin-related disorders in order to reduce damage and improve recovery, as well as the quality of life of these patients.

Chapter 1 – Oligodendrocytes have multiple functions in the central nervous system including mechanical support of neurons, production of myelin sheaths, and uptake and inactivation of chemical neurotransmitters released by neurons. Consequently, oligodendrocytes could be involved in the pathology of a number of neurodegenerative diseases. Although, the molecular mechanisms involved require further elucidation, it is likely that oligodendrocyte dysfunction is important in Alzheimer's disease (AD), amyotrophic lateral sclerosis (ALS), and multiple sclerosis (MS). In addition, abnormal protein aggregates in the form of oligodendrocyte inclusions (OI) have been observed in several other disorders, most notable in multiple system atrophy (MSA), in which the glial cytoplasmic inclusion (GCI) is the 'signature' pathology of the disease. OI have also been identified in argyrophilic grain disease (AGD), progressive supranuclear palsy (PSP), and various forms of frontotemporal lobar degeneration (FTLD) (Armstrong et al 2010), although their role in the pathology of these disorders is less clear. It is likely that future research will expand the range of disorders in which oligodendrocytes play a significant role in neurodegeneration.

Chapter 2 – Microglia have the potential for shaping the formation of new oligodendrocytes and controlling myelination and remyelination through direct and indirect mechanisms. Likewise, oligodendrocytes have functions that go beyond myelin production and extend to modulating microglial behavior and activation. Here, the authors review the effects of microglia on oligodendrocytes in both physiological and pathological conditions. The authors focus on the outcomes of the microglia-oligodendrocyte interaction in terms of myelination, oligodendrocyte differentiation, oligodendrocyte death, and remyelination while highlighting the influence of the activation state of microglia on the outcome of such interactions.

Chapter 3 – The myelin sheath that is formed by oligodendrocytes (OLs) insulate the axon from electrical activity and allow the rapid conduction of nerve impulses across axons. Direct mechanical injury and pathophysiological changes in secondary injury to the spinal cord cause death of OLs and demyelination of axons. Oligodendrocyte precursors (OPCs) maintain their capability of continuous generation throughout life. The adult central nervous system retains the potential to generate OPCs and the capacity for myelination after spinal cord injury (SCI). OPCs migrate from gray and white matter to the lesion, and after SCI, they differentiate into OLs that eventually myelinate axons. However, the intrinsic capacity for remyelination by OPCs is limited in the adult spinal cord. Focal delivery of cells, including OPCs, OPCs derived from embryonic stem cells (ECSs) and neural stem cells (NSCs), Schwann cells (SCs), and olfactory-ensheathing cells (OECs), has been investigated to remyelinate axons and promote functional recovery. A biomaterial scaffold that mediates the contact guidance of neural tissue growth and provides a permissive microenvironment for grafted cell growth can act as a vehicle for cell delivery in order to enhance axonal myelination. Improvement of cell transplantation strategies is a promising approach for the effective treatment of SCI clinically.

Chapter 4 – Oligodendrocytes (OL) are the main target of the pathological process during Multiple Sclerosis (MS). OL death and demyelination are constantly observed in MS lesions, together with axon damage and decrease in axon cytoskeleton protein (neurofilaments, tubulin) expression. Remyelination may occur but is never complete, leading to permanent disability. Mature myelinating OL are the main cells of the OL lineage in the adult central nervous system (CNS) and may participate, together with OL progenitors (OLP) in lesion repair. However, the capacity of these cells to survive insults, to grow new processes, and to synthesize new myelin sheaths is partly unknown. The molecules driving this phenomenon have not been deciphered yet. The authors review some of our data showing the induction of some plasticity of OL by growth factors and axon proteins *in vitro*. Restricted plasticity also was observed *in vivo*, in murine demyelinating lesions, and in MS lesions.

Despite the fact that mature myelinating OL represent the ultimate differentiation stage of OL development, *in vitro* some growth factors such as basic fibroblast growth factor (bFGF) are able to induce partial dedifferentiation of the cells with decreased myelin basic protein (MBP) expression and synthesis of loose myelin membranes (Fressinaud et al., 1995). Using lysophosphatidyl choline (LPC) as a toxic demyelinating agent, it was also observed that either bFGF or platelet-derived growth factor (PDGF) increase OL survival and synthesis of new myelin membranes *in vitro*. Similarly unique demyelinating events in rat demyelinating paradigm result in complete remyelination, and single stereotactic injection of growth factors (PDGF, neurotrophin-3 (NT-3)) accelerate this repair. However MS often occurs in a remittent-relapsing course and remyelination fails. The capacity of OL to survive multiple insults was demonstrated to be diminished *in vitro* with our LPC model, even in the presence of growth factors. This was akin to analysis of OL and myelinated fibers in MS lesions compared to the adjacent normal appearing white matter. As could be expected the number of OL was decreased in MS lesions, moreover the number of myelinated fibers per cell was decreased even more. Similar results were obtained with LPC lesions *in vivo* since controls (incomplete remyelination) showed a lower number of myelinated fibers per OL than NT-3-treated animals (robust remyelination).

Axons, which undergo degenerative changes during demyelination, are one of the main partners of OL; however, their crosstalk is poorly identified. The authors have shown that, following LPC and PDGF injection, remyelination alleviates these axonal lesions with an increase in NF expression in the rat model. Nevertheless, a striking event during MS is the release of NF and tubulin (TUB) in the cerebrospinal fluid, probably as a result of axon lesions. However, the role of NF when they are outside from the axon was unknown. They observed that NF, and other cytoskeleton proteins from the axon, as well as synthetic peptides corresponding to specific NF sequences increase OL growth, and differentiation. In addition, these proteins and peptides increase OL survival and partially protect them from LPC toxicity *in vitro*. Thus, these proteins could participate *in vivo* in a subtle bidirectional crosstalk with OL. So, extracellular NF could favorize OL plasticity and myelin repair, whereas in return remyelination could promote axon regeneration.

Chapter 5 – S100B, a Ca^{2+}-binding protein, is expressed mainly by astrocytes and maturing oligodendrocytes within the central nervous system (CNS). Intracellular S100B stimulates cell proliferation and migration, while at the extracellular level engages a few receptors with different outcomes depending on concentration, cell type and microenvironment. In the CNS, S100B promotes neuroprotection at low levels but if highly expressed may increase glial reactivity and induce brain damage. Although the effects of S100B on astrocytes, microglia and immune cells have been highly explored, only a few more recent reports implicate S100B in oligodendrocyte physiology and pathology. Here the authors describe S100 proteins, the intracellular and extracellular effect of S100B on CNS cells, namely in oligodendrogenesis, and its involvement in myelin-related disorders. Furthermore, they highlight the association of increased S100B concentration in the serum and cerebrospinal fluid of patients suffering from myelin-related disorders and shed some light on the mechanisms of S100B-induced myelin injury. Finally, the authors discuss the potential use of anti-S100B therapies to treat these disorders in order to reduce damage and improve recovery, as well as the quality of life of these patients.

In: Oligodendrocytes
Editor: Dana Swanson

ISBN: 978-1-63483-330-1

Chapter 1

Oligodendrocyte Pathology in Neurodegenerative Disease

Richard A. Armstrong*
Vision Sciences, Aston University, Birmingham, UK

Abstract

Oligodendrocytes have multiple functions in the central nervous system including mechanical support of neurons, production of myelin sheaths, and uptake and inactivation of chemical neurotransmitters released by neurons. Consequently, oligodendrocytes could be involved in the pathology of a number of neurodegenerative diseases. Although, the molecular mechanisms involved require further elucidation, it is likely that oligodendrocyte dysfunction is important in Alzheimer's disease (AD), amyotrophic lateral sclerosis (ALS), and multiple sclerosis (MS). In addition, abnormal protein aggregates in the form of oligodendrocyte inclusions (OI) have been observed in several other disorders, most notable in multiple system atrophy (MSA), in which the glial cytoplasmic inclusion (GCI) is the 'signature' pathology of the disease. OI have also been identified in argyrophilic grain disease (AGD), progressive supranuclear palsy (PSP) (Armstrong et al 2007), and various forms of

* Corresponding Author: Dr. R.A. Armstrong, Vision Sciences, Aston University, Birmingham, B4 7ET, UK. Tel 0121-359-3611, Fax 0121-333-4220, EMail: R.A.Armstrong@aston.ac.uk.

frontotemporal lobar degeneration (FTLD) (Armstrong et al 2010), although their role in the pathology of these disorders is less clear. It is likely that future research will expand the range of disorders in which oligodendrocytes play a significant role in neurodegeneration.

Keywords: oligodendrocyte, oligodendrocyte inclusion (OI), Alzheimer's disease (AD), amyotrophic lateral sclerosis (ALS), multiple sclerosis (MS), multiple system atrophy (MSA)

Introduction

In histological sections of brain tissue, the majority of nuclei visible in conventional Nissl or haematoxylin and eosin (H/E) stained preparations are glial cells (literally 'glue cells') (Glees, 1955; Kuffler and Nicholls, 1984), these nuclei being up to ten times more numerous than neurons (Nauta and Fiertag, 1986). The cell bodies of glial cells are not visible in Nissl-stained sections as there are insufficient ribosomes in the cytoplasm to bind the Nissl dye. Various functions have been ascribed to glial cells including mechanical support of neurons, production of the myelin sheaths around axons, the uptake and inactivation of chemical neurotransmitters released by neurons, the formation of scar tissue after injury, the removal of local tissue debris after death, as a filtration system between blood and neurons, and in the regulation of the extracellular fluid (Bradford, 1986).

Types of Glial Cell

There are three main types of glial cell visible in Nissl and H/E preparations of brain tissue (Figure 1). The largest lighter-staining nuclei have an irregular cell body and numerous processes that radiate outwards, thus resembling the appearance of a star, and are called astrocytes. These cells essentially form a matrix or 'scaffolding' in which the neurons are embedded. In addition, superficial astrocytes send their processes to the surface of the brain where the aggregation of their 'end feet' form a limiting membrane, viz., a 'glial capsule' constituting the outer wall of the brain and spinal cord by fusing with the pia mater and forming the pial-glial membrane. Where blood vessels from the surface penetrate brain tissue as the vertically penetrating arterioles, the pial-glial membrane also invaginates to follow the course of these vessels, thus constituting a component of the blood brain barrier (BBB). The second type of cell, appearing as small darkly-stained round nuclei, is the oligodendrocyte, strictly 'glial cell with few processes'. Oligodendrocytes coat axons in brain and spinal cord with lipid and protein, essentially forming the myelin sheaths. Hence, the oligodendroglial membrane compacts on itself to form approximately 40 veil-like extrusions, each consisting of a double membrane, and which wrap around the axon, more of these layers being added as the axon grows. The third type of glial cell in the central nervous system is the microglia, in which the nucleus is also dark but less regular in shape, often having an angular appearance. Microglia may not originate within the central nervous system but to arrive in association with the invaginating blood vessels during brain development.

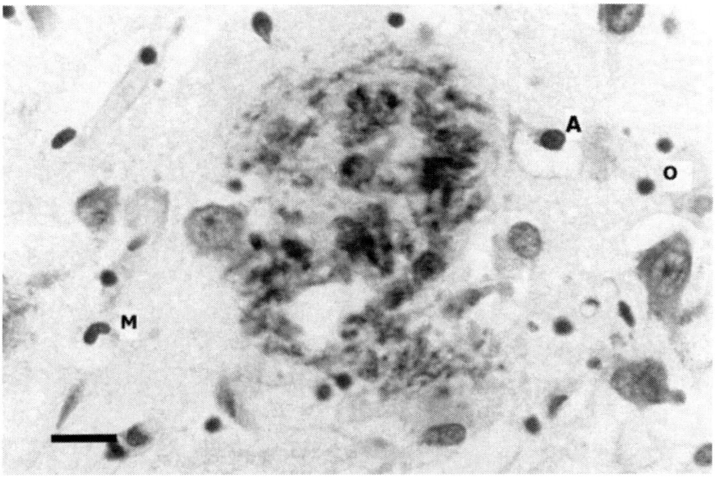

Figure 1. Glial cells (A = Astrocyte nucleus, O = Oligodendrocyte nucleus, M = Microglia nucleus) associated with a β-amyloid (Aβ) deposit in a case of Alzheimer's disease (AD) ($A\beta_{1-42}$ immunohistochemistry, Haematoxylin; Bar = 10 μm).

Development of Oligodendrocytes

Oligodendrocytes develop from precursor cells which can be identified by the expression of various antigens including ganglioside GD3, NG2 chondroitin sulphate proteoglycan, and platelet-derived growth factor (Pringle et al., 1992). These cells originate in the ventricular zone of the embryonic spinal cord and possibly the forebrain (Richardson et al., 2006) and are the last type of cell to be formed in the central nervous system (Thomas et al., 2000). Myelination by oligodendrocytes only occurs in relatively few brain regions at birth but continues into adulthood, a process which is not completed until 25-30 years of age (Fields, 2008). In adult brain, however, oligodendrocytes are formed in association with oligodendrocyte progenitor cells (OPG) (Menn et al., 2006). These cells migrate from the germinal zone to populate white and gray matter where they differentiate into mature myelin-forming oligodendrocytes. In addition, some oligodendrocytes may undergo apoptosis, while others fail to differentiate into mature cells and persist in the tissue as progenitor cells.

Types of Oligodendrocyte

There are at least three types of oligodendrocyte present in human brain (Figure 2). First, 'satellite' oligodendrocytes (SO) are found close to neuronal membranes in gray matter. These oligodendrocytes, which are not attached directly to neurons, do not serve an insulating role and are functionally distinct from the other types. The likely function of the SO is to regulate the composition of the extracellular fluid and especially the level of potassium (Baumann and Pham-Dinh, 2001). Second, occasional oligodendrocytes with perivascular attachments, known as vascular oligodendrocytes (VO), can be observed in gray matter adjacent to capillaries. Third, interfascicular oligodendrocytes (IO) are found in white matter and responsible for myelin formation in the central nervous system and therefore, are the counterpart of Schwann cells found in the peripheral nervous system. A single oligodendrocyte can extend its processes around 50 axons, wrapping approximately 1 μm of myelin around each axon.

Oligodendrocytes and Disease

Activation of glial cells in brain, mainly astrocytes and microglia, as a result of disease ('gliosis') is important in the pathology of several neurodegenerative diseases (Mena and Garcia de Yebenés, 2008; Heneka et al., 2010; Singh et al., 2011). Significantly less attention has been paid to oligodendrocytes, however, as they were believed to be largely myelin-forming cells and therefore, only likely to be involved in demyelinating disease. However, injury to oligodendrocytes occurs in several nervous system diseases, not only in demyelinating diseases such as multiple sclerosis (MS) and the various leukodystrophies where, for example, they are susceptible to JC virus as in progressive multifocal leukoencephalopathy (PML), but also in trauma and cerebral palsy. Oligodendrocyte damage has also been implicated in such disorders as schizophrenia and bipolar disorder (Tkachev et al., 2003).

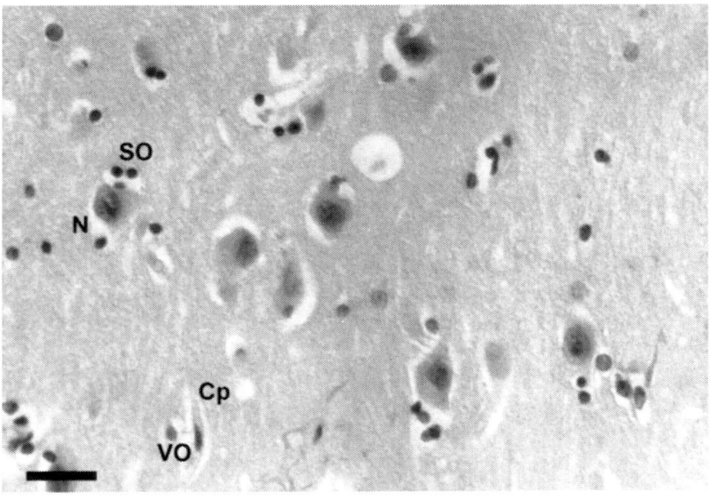

Figure 2. Types of oligodendrocyte observed in gray matter of the human brain (SO = Satellite oligodendrocyte, VO = Vascular oligodendrocyte, Cp = Capillary, N = Neuronal cell body (H/E, Bar = 10 μm).

As oligodendrocytes support neurons and their axons (Nave and Trapp, 2008; Nave et al., 2010a; 2010b), they could be involved in various pathogenic processes. First, damage to oligodendrocytes can result in the loss of intact myelin sheaths and therefore, play a direct role in MS and the leukodystrophies (Feigenbaum et al., 2000). Hence, in animal models of disease, oligodendrocytes are necessary for axon integrity under physiological conditions (Ghosh et al., 2011; Pohl et al., 2011; Oluich et al., 2012). Oligodendrocytes also support axons and maintain functional integrity as a result of various mechanisms other than myelination (Nave, 2010a; 2010b; Nave and Trapp, 2008). Second, metabolic coupling between oligodendrocytes and neurons is important for neuronal survival and hence, disruption of this process could contribute to neurodegeneration (Liu and Zhou, 2013). Third, oligodendrocytes could be involved in the formation and subsequent growth of abnormal protein deposits in brain such as β-amyloid (Aβ) in Alzheimer's disease (AD) and the disease form of prion protein (PrP^{sc}) in Creutzfeldt-Jakob disease (CJD) and in both disorders, in the evolution of early diffuse-type deposits to more mature plaques (Armstrong et al., 2003). Abnormal protein aggregates in the form of deposits could also damage adjacent oligodendrocytes as well as neurons thus influencing further the processes of myelination and extracellular fluid regulation. Fourth, oligodendrocytes could be involved in attempts to remove abnormal proteins from the brain resulting in their accumulation within the cell in the form of oligodendrocyte inclusions (OI). One of the most significant pathologies of this type is the glial cytoplasmic inclusion (GCI) observed in multiple system atrophy (MSA) (Papp et al., 1989). Fifth, damage to VO may contribute to a disruption of the BBB in neurodegenerative disease contributing further to the deposition of abnormal proteins within the brain.

Hence, the objective of this chapter is to examine the role that oligodendrocytes may play in a variety of neurodegenerative disease with special reference to AD, amyotrophic lateral sclerosis (ALS), MS, and MSA.

Oligodendrocytes and Neurodegenerative Disease

Alzheimer's Disease (AD)

AD is a degenerative disorder of the nervous system affecting approximately 10% of individuals aged 65 or over (Knopman, 2001). The development of dementia in AD involves a decline in short-term memory, impairment of judgment, and a loss of emotional control. These symptoms develop slowly over a period of years resulting ultimately in a complete breakdown of mental function. A small proportion of cases of AD (<5%) have a genetic origin but most cases occur sporadically within the population (Hoenicka, 2006). The pathology of AD includes the deposition in the brain of abnormal aggregates of Aβ in the form of extracellular senile plaques (SP) and intracellular phosphorylated tau-reactive neurofibrillary tangles (Armstrong, 2006).

Several sources of evidence implicate oligodendrocyte dysfunction in the neurodegeneration of AD. First, damage to oligodendrocytes has been observed as a result of brain aging (Sloane et al., 2003; Tanaka et al., 2005; Lasiene et al., 2009; Kohama et al., 2011), a major risk factor for AD

(Armstrong, 2013a). Second, the deposition of toxic isomers of Aβ in white matter of AD may cause axonal damage and the death of oligodendrocytes (Jantaratnotai et al., 2003; Lee et al., 2012; Desai et al., 2011).

In addition, increasing deposition of Aβ in white matter is often associated with a significant reduction of myelin basic protein (MBP) and the proteolipid protein (PLP), a product of a myelin-related gene with selective expression in oligodendrocytes and Schwann cells, and in 2'3'-cyclic nucleotide 3' phosphodiesterase (CNP1), processes which indicate white matter degeneration (Mitew et al., 2010). Supporting this hypothesis, axon loss has been observed in various white matter fibre tracts in AD including the optic nerve, olfactory tract, and corpus callosum (Syed et al., 2000) which could be due to a disorder which directly affects white matter. An associated white matter disorder linked to cerebrovascular disease has been reported in approximately 60% of patients with AD (Brun and Englund, 1986). This disorder is characterised by a loss of axons and oligodendrocytes, demyelination, and a mild reactive astrocytic gliosis. Third, development of oligodendrocytes may be protracted in those brain areas, such as the frontal and medial temporal lobes, which are most vulnerable to AD pathology (Bartzokis, 2004).

In addition, there is often extensive development of Aβ deposits in these regions in AD and oligodendrocytes are frequently observed adjacent to such deposits (Figure 1). Hence, damage to these oligodendrocytes may have further consequences for the integrity of adjacent neurons. Fourth, in transgenic mouse models of AD (Triple-Swedish model), alterations in myelin and in oligodendrocytes can be detected which precede the deposition of Aβ and tau (Desai et al., 2010).

Moreover, the presence of $A\beta_{1-42}$, a toxic isomer of Aβ, increases the expression of caspase-3 and apoptotic cell death in both non-differentiated and differentiated mouse oligodendrocyte precursors (Desai et al., 2010). It is also possible that oligodendrocytes are damaged in other disorders which are characterised by the deposition of extracellular toxic aggregated proteins, such as PrP^{sc} in CJD (Armstrong, 2013b).

Amyotrophic Lateral Sclerosis (ALS)

In amylotrophic lateral sclerosis (ALS), loss of upper and lower motor neurons results in problems with speaking, walking, breathing, swallowing, and in general movement of the body. Hence, ALS is closely related to other 'motor neuron-type' disorders such as spino-bulbar muscular atrophy, spinal muscular atrophy, and Charcot-Marie-Tooth disease. It was Charcot in 1869 who first suggested grouping together these various diseases which affect the lateral horn of the spinal cord as ALS. Approximately 90% of cases of ALS are sporadic and both genetic and environmental factors are likely to be involved in the aetiology of these cases. The 10% of familial cases have been associated with a variety of different genes including superoxide dismutase (*SOD1*), *ALS2*, senataxin (*SETX*), and vesicle-associated protein B (*VAPB*), *SOD1* being the most common gene associated with familial ALS. The neuropathology of ALS is characterized by the degeneration of the ventral horns of the spinal cord accompanied by atrophy of the ventral roots while in the cerebral cortex, there may be degeneration of frontal and temporal lobes. Histological features include vacuolation, astrocytosis, and skein-like cellular inclusions called 'Bunina bodies'.

The involvement of oligodendrocytes and their precursors has been implicated in both human patients with ALS and in animal models of the disease (Kang et al., 2013; Philips et al., 2013). Hence, oligodendrocyte dysfunction in human ALS can result in demyelination of gray matter and reactive changes in motor cortex and spinal cord (Kang et al., 2013). In addition, morphological changes in oligodendrocytes in gray matter are often apparent before disease onset, becoming more pronounced with disease progression, and followed by the death of these cells (Philips et al., 2013). Death of oligodendrocytes, however, is often compensated by increased proliferation and differentiation of oligodendrocyte precursors. Nevertheless, these newly differentiated oligodendrocytes are often dysfunctional and exhibit reductions in MBP and in various transporter molecules responsible for transferring glycolytic substrates to neurons and to oligodendrocyte precursors.

In addition, in animals that overexpress *SOD1*, the expression of transporter monocarboxylate transporter 1 protein was also reduced (Philips et al., 2013) and removal of this mutant gene from these cells delayed disease onset and prolonged survival. Hence, ALS-linked genes may enhance the vulnerability of motor neurons and accelerate disease by impairing oligodendrocyte function in ALS (Kang et al., 2013).

Multiple Sclerosis (MS)

Multiple sclerosis (MS), one of the commonest progressively disabling diseases to affect the young, was first described by Charcot in 1868. MS is rare in childhood, but after the age of 17, it increases in prevalence reaching a peak in the third decade of life. New cases occur but with decreasing frequency into the sixth decade (Armstrong, 1999). MS primarily affects myelin often leaving the axons intact (Adams, 1983; Gregson, 1983) and severe loss of myelin may occur at several sites in the nervous system, the result often completely blocking nerve conduction. Four sites are especially vulnerable in MS, viz., the optic nerves, the upper region of the spinal cord, brain stem, and cerebellum (Armstrong, 1999). MS is clinically variable and a typical course may include an initial attack followed by a complete recovery. New symptoms subsequently develop, usually after several months, and are again followed by recovery. Nevertheless, further relapses occur at intervals, and each time the recovery may be less complete so that eventually, persistent difficulties result.

MS is believed to be an inflammatory demyelinating disease associated with focal destruction of the myelin sheaths and astrocytic scar formation (Lumsden, 1970). Hence, the formation of discreet areas called 'sclerotic or demyelination plaques' is the major pathological feature observed in MS at post-mortem (Armstrong, 1999). In appearance, the plaques are sharply defined, grey-yellow, rubbery and semi-translucent areas which may vary in size and shape. The earliest detectable stage in development of a plaque appears to be the formation of a cluster of lymphocytes located around a small vein in brain or spinal cord. The lymphocytes spread along the vein and become associated with an area of tissue in which loss of myelin occurs. The plaque and surrounding regions became inflamed and swollen with excess fluid and there is an associated gliosis involving the proliferation of astrocytes and oligodendrocytes, followed by microglial phagocytosis. The oligodendrocytes are often abnormally enlarged and proliferate at the rim of the plaque but can also be distributed throughout active plaques. Initial hyperplasia of oligodendrocytes may be followed by the death of these cells (Adams, 1983) with consequent implications for remyelination (Harrison, 1983).

The sequence of events in MS leading to myelin breakdown and repair, including the fate of oligodendrocytes, is unclear (Luchinetti et al., 1999). Hence, injury to oligodendrocytes, either as a result of toxins, viruses (Meulen and Stephenson, 1983), or immune-mediated attack may lead to initial demyelination and contribute to the formation of the sclerotic plaque

(Lampert, 1983). A variety of possible immune-mediated mechanisms could damage oligodendrocytes in MS (Figure 3). First, direct T-cell mediated cytotoxicity could occur via the Fas-Fas ligand pathway (D'Souza et al., 1996; Dowling et al., 1996). Second, products of T-cells, such as perforin or lymphotoxins could directly damage oligodendrocytes (Scolding et al., 1990; Selmaj et al., 1999a,b). Third, activated macrophages, which release cytokines or reactive oxygen species (ROS), could be involved (Selmaj and Raine, 1988; Griot et al., 1990). Fourth, antibodies and/or complement proteins in serum could attack and damage oligodendrocytes (Bornstein and Appel, 1961; Brosnan et al., 1977).

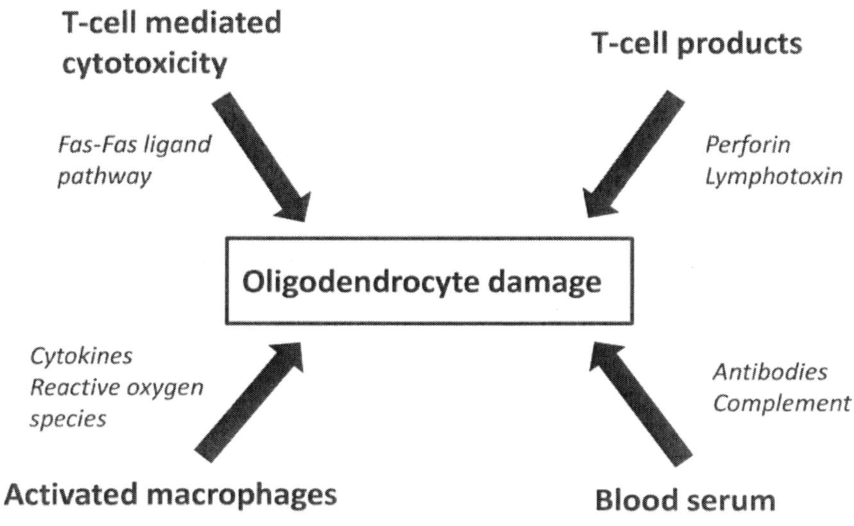

Figure 3. Mechanisms of immune-mediated damage to oligodendrocytes in multiple sclerosis (MS).

In older, more mature sclerotic plaques, oligodendrocytes are largely absent (Lumsden, 1970; Lassmann, 1983; Prineas, 1985) but variable numbers of these cells have been observed in actively developing lesions (Prineas, 1975; Raine et al., 1981; Lassman, 1983; Lucchinetti et al., 1996; Storch et al., 1988). In a quantitative study of a large number of patients, two groups of MS cases were identified (Lucchinetti et al., 1999). Hence, in the majority (comprising 70% of the sample), oligodendrocytes were variably reduced during the active stage of the plaque but reappeared within inactive plaques and in areas of remyelination.

In the remaining cases (30% of the sample), there was extensive destruction of myelin-forming cells at active sites and oligodendrocytes were absent in those inactive plaques which were not exhibiting remyelination. Hence, there may be subsets of MS patients in which myelin, mature oligodendrocytes, and possibly their progenitors are being differentially affected (Lucchinetti et al., 1999).

Multiple System Atrophy (MSA)

MSA is a relatively 'new' descriptive term derived from three previously described diseases, viz., olivopontocerebellar atrophy, striato-nigral degeneration, and Shy-Drager syndrome (Probst-Cousin et al., 2000). The symptoms of MSA include Parkinsonism, ataxia, and autonomic dysfunction (Lantos, 1994). Ataxia describes a gross lack of coordination of muscle movements while autonomic dysfunction involves a variety of systems that regulate unconscious bodily functions such as heart rate, blood pressure, bladder function, and digestion. The mean age of onset of MSA is 54.2 years (range 31 – 78 years) (Ben-Schlomo et al., 1997). The average annual incidence of the disorder is 3.0/100,000 of the population and the median survival time is 8.5 years, (Bower et al., 1997) an older age of onset being associated with a shorter survival time. The disorder is slightly more common in males than females (Male:Female ratio 1.3:1) and symptoms usually begin early in the fifth decade of life (Wenning et al., 1997).

Approximately 74% of MSA patients exhibit autonomic failure, 87% Parkinsonism, 54% cerebellar ataxia, and 49% pyramidal signs such as paralysis, muscle weakness, loss of muscle control, and tremor. The most consistent clinical syndrome in MSA is the presence of Parkinsonism, followed by autonomic dysfunction, cerebellar ataxia, and pyramidal tract signs (Wenning et al., 1997). Of the autonomic system problems, occurrence of urinary dysfunction is the more common symptom and an earlier manifestation of the disease than orthostatic hypotension (postural low blood pressure).

The most important visual signs include oculomotor dysfunction and pupil reactivity, but with relatively preserved primary vision. Patients with either predominantly cerebellar signs or Parkinsonism are regarded as distinct subtypes of MSA and designated as MSA-C and MSA-P respectively. Patients with cerebellar features have marginally increased survival times but the prognosis is poor for most patients. Patients with MSA-P often have abnormal movements of the hands and fingers referred to as a 'jerky' tremor or myoclonus. No abnormal movements are usually present at rest. When holding a posture, however, small amplitude, non-rhythmic movements of one or a few fingers may occur. There is a moderate intellectual impairment in some patients but severe loss of cognitive function or dementia is unusual (Wenning et al., 1997).

Oligodendrocyte dysfunction may contribute to both disease initiation and progression of MSA (Kahle et al., 2002; Ozawa et al., 2004; Shults et al., 2005; Sternberger et al., 2010). The most characteristic pathological change observed in MSA is the presence of abnormal protein aggregates, termed glial cytoplasmic inclusions (GCI), found mainly in oligodendrocytes, and first described in 1989 (Papp et al., 1989) (Figure 4). The GCI comprise abnormal aggregations of silver-positive, 10-15 nm diameter coated filaments, the major molecular constituent of which is the protein α-synuclein. A significant correlation between the frequency of GCI in MSA and the severity of neuronal loss and disease duration has been demonstrated (Liu and Zhou, 2013). In addition, overexpression of α-synuclein in oligodendrocytes decreases glial-derived neurotrophic factor (GDNF) levels *in vivo* and *in vitro* (Ubhi et al., 2010), reductions in GDNF also being observed in brain tissue of MSA patients. The accumulation of pathogenic α-synuclein in these cells may be a precursor to the death of oligodendrocytes with consequences for remyelination and neuronal integrity.

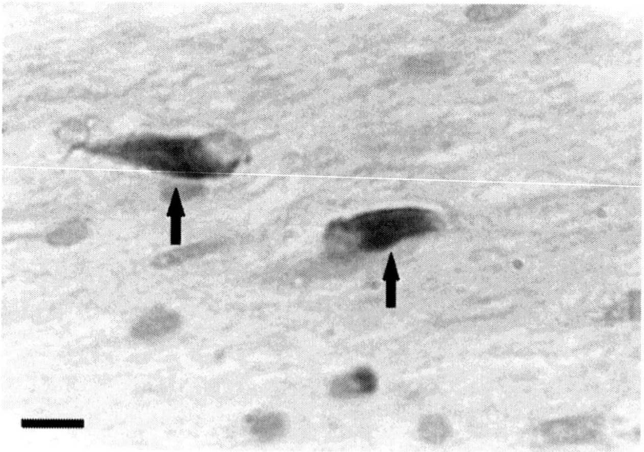

Figure 4. Glial cytoplasmic inclusions (GCI) (arrows) in cerebellar white matter in a case of multiple system atrophy (MSA) (α-synuclein immunohistochemistry, Bar = 6 μm).

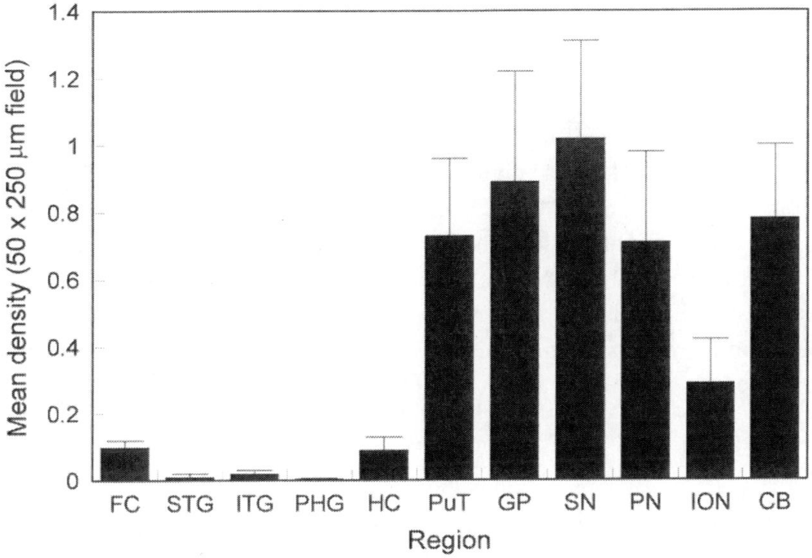

Figure 5. Mean density of glial cytoplasmic inclusions (GCI) in various brain regions (PuT = Putamon, GP = Globus pallidus, SN = Substantia nigra, PN = Pons PN, ION = Inferior olivary nucleus, CB = Cerebellar hemisphere, FC = Frontal cortex, STG = Superior temporal gyrus, ITG = Inferior temporal gyrus, PHG = Parahippocampal gyrus, HC = Hippocampus) in multiple system atrophy (MSA). Data from Armstrong et al., (2004). Error bars indicate SE of mean.

The greatest densities of GCI are often seen in basal ganglia (Figure 5) including the putamen (PT), globus pallidus (GP), and substantia nigra (SN). Significant numbers of GCI can also be observed in the pons (PN), inferior olivary nucleus (ION), and cerebellum hemisphere (CB). Relatively low densities of GCI, however, are observed in the superior frontal gyrus (SFG), superior temporal gyrus (STG), inferior temporal gyrus (ITG), parahippocampal gyrus (PHG), and hippocampus (HC). Hence, oligodendrocyte dysfunction in MSA is likely to significantly affect subcortical rather than cortical regions.

Other Neurodegenerative Diseases

Abnormal aggregations of pathological proteins in the form of OI have been reported in a variety of other neurodegenerative disorders but their role in the pathology of these diseases is unclear. Hence, phosphorylated tau-reactive

OI have been observed as a common additional finding in argyrophilic grain disease (AGD) (Braak and Braak, 1998) and in various forms of frontotemporal lobar degeneration (FTLD) including corticobasal degeneration (CBD), FTLD with TDP-43-reactive inclusions (FTLD-TDP) (Armstrong et al., 2010), and neuronal intermediate filament inclusion disease (NIFID) (Armstrong et al., 2011). In addition, GI, together with other forms of glial pathology are a feature of the pathology of progressive supranuclear palsy (PSP) especially in subcortical motor areas such as the striatum, substantia nigra, red nucleus, locus caeruleus, pons, and inferior olivary nucleus (Armstrong et al., 2007) (Fig 6). In most of these disorders, the role of glial pathology in the disease and its relationship to neuronal pathology remains to be elucidated.

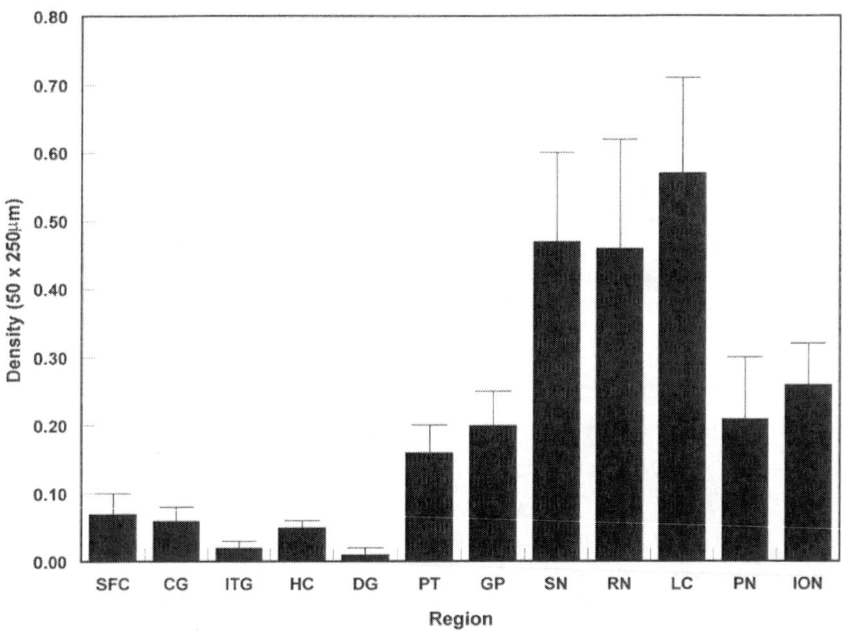

Figure 6. Mean density of oligodendrocyte inclusions (OI) in various brain regions (PT = Putamon, GP = Globus pallidus, SN = Substantia nigra, PN = Pons, ION = Inferior olivary nucleus, RN = Red nucleus, LC = Locus careuleus, SFC = Superior frontal cortex, CG = Cingulate gyrus, ITG = Inferior temporal gyrus, HC = Hippocampus, DG = Dentate gyrus) in progressive supranuclear palsy (PSP). Data from Armstrong et al., (2007). Error bars indicate SE of mean.

Conclusion

Oligodendrocytes have multiple functions in the central nervous system including mechanical support of neurons, production of the myelin sheaths around axons, the uptake and inactivation of chemical neurotransmitters released by neurons and are therefore, likely to be important in a number of neurodegenerative diseases. Although, the molecular mechanisms involved in neurodegeneration require further elucidation, it is likely that oligodendrocyte dysfunction plays an important role in AD, ALS, MS, and MSA. In addition, OI have been observed in several additional diseases including AGD, PSP (Armstrong et al., 2007), and various forms of FTLD (Armstrong et al., 2010) and further research is likely to expand the range of disorders in which oligodendrocytes may play a significant role in neurodegeneration.

References

Adams CWM. General pathology of multiple sclerosis. In: *Multiple Sclerosis*. Ed: Hallpike JF, Adams CWM & Tourtellotte WW. Williams & Wilkins, Baltimore, 1983, 203-240.

Armstrong RA. Multiple sclerosis and the eye. *Ophthal. Physiol. Opt.* 1999, 19, S32-S42.

Armstrong RA. Plaques and tangles and the pathology of Alzheimer's disease. *Folia Neuropathol* 2006, 44, 1-11.

Armstrong RA. What causes Alzheimer's disease? *Folia Neuropathol.* 2013a, 51, 169-188.

Armstrong RA. Glia and the pathology of variant Creutzfeldt-Jakob disease (vCJD). In: *Glial cells: Embryonic development, Types/Functions and Role in Disease*. (Ed. C. Kaur, Ang LE), Nova Science Publishers, 2013b, 89-106.

Armstrong RA, Lantos PL, Ironside JW, Cairns NJ. Differences in the density and spatial distribution of florid and diffuse plaques in variant Creutzfeldt-Jakob disease (vCJD). *Clin. Neuropathol.* 2003, 22, 209-214.

Armstrong RA, Lantos PL, Cairns NJ. Progressive supranuclear palsy (PSP: a quantitative study of the pathological changes in cortical and subcortical regions of eight cases. *J. Neural. Transm.* 2007, 114, 1569-1577.

Armstrong RA, Ellis W, Hamilton RL, Mackenzie IRA, Hedreen J, Gearing M, Montine T, Vonsattel J-P, Head E, Lieberman AP, Cairns NJ.

Neuropathological heterogeneity in frontotemporal lobar degeneration with TDP-43 proteinopathy: a quantitative study of 94 cases using principal components analysis. *J. Neural. Transm.* 2010; 117: 227-239.

Armstrong RA, Gearing M, Bigio EH, Cruz-Sanchez FF, Duyckaerts C, Mackenzie IRA, Perry RH, Skullerud K, Yokoo H, Cairns NJ. The spectrum and severity of FUS-immunoreactive inclusions in frontal and temporal lobes of ten cases on neuronal intermediate filament inclusion disease. *Acta. Neuropathol.* 2011, 121, 219-228.

Bartzokis G. Age-related myelin breakdown: a developmental model of cognitive decline and Alzheimer's disease. *Neurobiol. Aging* 2004, 5, 5-18.

Baumann N, Pham-Dinh D. Biology of oligodendrocyte and myelin in the mammalian central nervous sytem. *Physiol. Rev.* 2001, 18, 871-927.

Ben-Shlomo Y, Wenning GK, Tison F, Quinn NP. Survival of patients with pathologically proven multiple system atrophy: A meta-analysis. *Neurology* 1997, 48, 384-393.

Bornstein MB, Appel SH. The application of tissue culture to the study of experimental 'allergic' encephalomyelitis. I. Patterns of demyelination. *J. Neuropathol. Exp. Neurol.* 1961, 20, 141-147.

Bower JH, Maraganore DM, McDonnell K, Rocca WA. Incidence of progressive supranuclear palsy and multiple system atrophy in Olmstead County, Minnesota, 1976-1990. *Neurology* 1997, 49, 1284-1288.

Braak H, Braak E. Argyrophilic grain disease: Frequency of occurrence in different age categories and neuropathologic diagnostic criteria. *J. Neural. Transm.* 1998, 105, 801-819.

Bradford HF. *Chemical neurobiology: An Introduction to Neurochemistry*. WF Freeman and Co., New York, 1986.

Brosnan CF, Stoner GL, Bloom BR, Wisniewski HM. Studies on demyelination by activated lymphocytes in the rabbit eye. II. Antibody-dependent cell-mediated demyelination. *J. Immunol.* 1977, 118, 2103-2110.

Brun A and Englund E. A white matter disorder in dementia of the Alzheimer type: a patho-anatomical study. *Ann. Neurol.* 1986, 19, 253-262.

D'Souza SD, Bonetti B, Balasingam V, Cashman NR, Barker PA. Troutt AB et al., Multiple sclerosis: Fas signalling in oligodendrocyte cell death. *J. Exp. Med.* 1996, 184, 2361-2370.

Desai MK, Mastrangelo MA, Ryan DA, Sudol KL, Narrow WC, Bowers WJ. Early oligodendrocyte/myelin pathology in Alzheimer's disease mice constitutes a novel therapeutic target. *Am. J. Pathol.* 2010, 177, 1422-1435.

Desai MK, Guercio BJ, Narrow WC, Bowers WJ. An Alzheimer's disease-relevant presenilin-1 mutation augments amyloid-beta-induced oligodendrocyte dysfunction. *Glia* 2011, 59, 627-640.

Dowling P, Shang G, Raval S, Menonna J, Cook S, Husar W. Involvement of the CD94 (APO-1/Fas) receptor/ligand system in multiple sclerosis brain. *J. Exp. Med.* 1996, 184, 1513-1568.

Feigenbaum V, Gélot A, Casanova P, Daumas-Duport C, Aubourg P, Dubois-Daleq M. Apoptosis in the central nervous system of cerebral adrenoleukodystrophy patients. *Neurobiol. Dis.* 2000, 7, 600-612.

Fields D. White matter matters. *Scientific American* 2008, 298, 54-61.

Ghosh A, Manrique-Hoyos N, Voigt A, Schultz JB, Kreutzfeld M, Merkler D, Simons M. Targated ablation of oligodendrocytes triggers axonal damage. *PLoS ONE* 2011, 6, e22735.

Glees P. *Neuroglia Morphology and Function*. Thomas, Springfield, Ill, 1955.

Gregson NA. The molecular biology of myelin. In: *Multiple Sclerosis*. Ed: Hallpike JF, Adams CWM & Tourtellotte WW. Williams & Wilkins, Baltimore, 1983, 1-28.

Griot C, Vandevelde M, Richard A, Peterhans E, Stocker R. Selective degeneration of oligodendrocytes mediated by reactive oxygen species. *Free Rad. Res. Commun.* 1990, 11, 181-193.

Harrison BM. Remyelination in the central nervous system. In: *Multiple Sclerosis*. Ed: Hallpike JF, Adams CWM & Tourtellotte WW. Williams & Wilkins, Baltimore, 1983, 461-478.

Heneka MT, Rodriguez JJ, Verkhatsky A. Neuroglia in neurodegeneration. *Brain Res. Rev.* 2010, 63, 189-211.

Hoenicka J. Genes in Alzheimer's disease. *Rev de Neurol* 2006, 42, 302-305.

Kahle PJ, Neumann M, Oxmen L, Muller V, Jacobsen H, Spooren W, Fuss B, Mallon B, Macklin WB, Fujiwara H, Hasegawa M, Iwatsubo T, Kretzschmar HA, Haass C. Hyperphosphorylation and insolubility of alpha-synuclein in transgenic mouse oligodendrocytes. *EMBO rep* 2002, 3, 583-588.

Jantaratnotai N, Ryu JK, Kim SU, McLarnon JG. Amyloid beta peptide-induced corpus callosum damage and glial activation in vivo. *Neuroreport* 2003, 14, 1429-1433.

Kang SH, Ying L, Fukaya M, lorenzini DW, Ostrow LW, Rothstein JD, Bergles DE. Degeneration and impaired regeneration of gray matter oligodendrocytes in amyotrophic lateral sclerosis. *Nature Neurosci.* 2013, 16, 571-579.

Knopman DS. An overview of common non-Alzheimer dementias. *Clinics in Ger. Med.* 2001, 17, 281.

Kohama SG, Rosene DL, Sherman LS. Age-related changes in human and non-human primate white matter: from myelination disturbances to cognitive decline. *Age* 2011, 34, 1093-1110.

Kuffler SW, Nicholls JG. *From Neuron to Brain.* 2nd Ed., Sinauer, Sunderland, Mass., 1984.

Lampert PW. Fine structure of the demyelinating process. In: *Multiple Sclerosis.* Ed: Hallpike JF, Adams CWM & Tourtellotte WW. Williams & Wilkins, Baltimore, 1983, 20-46.

Lantos PL. Cellular pathology of multiple system atrophy: a review. *J. Neurol. Neurosurg. Psych.* 1994, 57, 129-13.

Lasiene J, Matsui A, Sawa Y, Wong F, Horner PJ. Age-related myelin dynamics revealed by increased oligodendrogenesis and short internodes. *Aging Cell* 2009, 8, 201-213.

Lassmann H. Comparataive neuropathology of chronic experimental allergic encephalomyelitis and multiple sclerosis. *Schriftnr. Neurol.* 1983, 25, 1-135.

Lee Y, Morrison BM, Lengacher S, Farah MH, Hoffman PN, Liu Y, Tsingalia A, Jin L, Zhang PW, Pellerin L, Magistretti PJ, Rothstein JD. Oligodendroglia metabolically support axons and contribute to neurodegeneration. *Nature* 2012, 487, 443-448.

Liu Y, Zhou, J. Oligodendrocytes in neurodegenerative diseases. *Front Biol.* 2013, 8, 127-133.

Lucchinetti CF, Brück W, Rodriguez M, Lassman H. Distinct patterns of multiple sclerosis pathology indicates heterogeneity on pathogenesis. *Brain Pathol.* 1996, 6, 259-274.

Lucchinetti C, Brück W, Parisi J, Scheithauer B, Rodriguez M, Lassman H. A quantitative analysis of oligodendrocytes in multiple sclerosis lesions: A study of 113 cases. *Brain* 1999, 122, 2279-2295.

Lumsden CE. The neuropathology of multiple sclerosis. In: Vinken PJ, Bruyn GW Eds., *Handbook of Clinical Neurology.* Amsterdam, North Holland 1970, 9, 217-309.

Mena MA, García de Yebenés J. Glial cells as players in parkinsonism: the 'good', the 'bad', and the 'mysterious' glia. *Neuroscientist* 2008, 14, 544-560.

Menn B, Garcia-Verdugo JM, Yaschine C, Gonzalez-Perez O, Rowitch D, Alvarez-Buylla A. Origin of oligodendrocytes in the subventricular zone of the adult brain. *J. Neurosci.* 2006, 26, 7907-7918.

Meulen V, Stephenson JR. The possible role of viral infections in multiple sclerosis and other related demyelinating diseases. In: *Multiple Sclerosis.* Ed: Hallpike JF, Adams CWM & Tourtellotte WW. Williams & Wilkins, Baltimore, 1983, 241-274.

Mitew S, Kirkcaldie MT, Halliday GM, Shepherd CE, Vickers JC, Dickson TC. Focal demyelination in Alzheimer's disease and transgenic mouse models. *Acta. Neuropathol.* 2010, 119, 567-577.

Nauta WJH, Feirtag M. *Fundamental Neuroanatomy.* WH Freeman & Co., New York, 1986.

Nave K. Myelination and support of axonal integrity by glia. *Nature* 2010a, 468, 244-252.

Nave KA. Myelination and the trophic support of long axons. *Nat. Rev. Neurosci.* 2010b, 11, 275-283.

Nave KA, Trapp BD. Axon-glial signalling and the glial support of axon function. *Ann. Rev. Neurosci.* 2008, 31, 535-561.

Oluich LJ, Stratton JA, Xing YL, Ng SW, Cate HS, Sah P, Windels F, Kilpatrick TJ, Merson TD. Targeted ablation of oligodendrocytes induces axonal pathology independent of overt demyelination. *J. Neurosci.* 2012, 32, 8317-8330.

Ozawa T, Paviour D, Quinn NP, Josephs KA, Sangha H, Kilford L, Healy DG, Wood NW, Lees AJ, Holton JL, Revesz T. The spectrum of pathological involvement of the striatonigral and olivopontocerebellar systems in multiple system atrophy: clinic-pathological correlations. *Brain* 2004, 127, 2657-2671.

Papp MI, Kahn JE, Lantos PL. Glial cytoplasmic inclusions in the CNS of patients with multiple system atrophy (striatonigral degeneration, olivopontocerebellar atrophy and Shy-Drager syndrome). *J. Neurol. Sci.* 1989; 94: 79-100.

Philips T, Bento-Abreu A, Nonneman A, Haek W, Staats K, Geelen V, Hersmus N, Kusters B, Bosch L Van D, Damme P Van, Richardson WD, Robberecht W. Oligodendrocyte dysfunction in the pathogenesis of amyotrophic lateral sclerosis. *Brain* 2013, 136, 471-482.

Pohl HB, Porcheri C, Mueggler T, Bachmann LC, Martino G, Riethmacher D, Franklin RJ, Rudin M, Suter U. Genetically induced adult oligodendrocyte cell death is associated with poor myelin clearance, reduced remyelination, and axonal damage. *J. Neurosci.* 2011, 31, 1069-1080.

Prineas J. Pathology of the early lesion in multiple sclerosis. *Hum. Pathol.* 1975, 6, 531-554.

Pringle NP, Mudhar HS, Collarini EJ, Richardson WD. PDGF receptors in the rat CNS: during late neurogenesis, PDGF alpha-receptor expression appears to be restricted to glial cells of the oligodendrocyte lineage. *Development* 1992, 115, 535-551.

Probst-Cousin S, Kayser C, Heuss D, Neundorfer B. Thirty years of multiple system atrophy concept: Review and survey of multiple system atrophy. *Fortschritte Neurol. Psych.* 2000, 68, 25-36.

Raine CS, Scheinberg L, Waltz JM. Multiple sclerosis: oligodendrocyte survival and proliferation in an active extablished lesion. *Lab. Invest.* 1981, 45, 534-546.

Richardson WD, Kessaris N, Pringle N. Oligodendrocyte wars. *Nature Rev.: Neurosci* 2006, 7, 8-11.

Scolding N, Jones J, Compston DA, Morgan BP. Oligodendrocyte susceptibility to injury by T-cell perforin. *Immunology* 1990, 70, 6-10.

Selmaj KW, Raine CS. Tumor necrosis factor mediates myelin and oligodendrocyte damage in vitro. *Ann. Neurol.* 1988, 23, 339-346.

Selmaj KW, Raine CS, Cannella B, Brosnan CF. Identification of lymphotoxin and tumor necrosis factor in multiple sclerosis lesions. *J. Clin. Invest.* 1991a, 87, 949-954.

Selmaj K, Raine CS, Farooq M, Norton WT, Brosman CF. Cytokine cytotoxicity against oligodendrocytes. Apoptosis induced by lymphotoxin. *J. Immunol.* 1991b, 147, 1522-1529.

Shults CW, Rockenstein E, Crewe L, Adams A, Mante M, Larrea G, Hashimoto M, Song D, Iwatsubo T, Tsuboi K, Masliah E. Neurological and neurodegenerative alterations in a transgenic mouse model expressing human alpha-synuclein under oligodendrocyte promotor: implications for multiple system atrophy. *J. Neurosci.* 2005, 25, 10689-10699.

Singh S, Swarnkar JD, Goswami P, Nath C. Astrocytes and microglia: responses to neuropathological conditions. *Int. J. Neurosci.* 2011, 121, 589-597.

Sloane JA, Hinman JD, Lubonia M, Hollander W, Abraham CR. Age-dependent myelin degeneration and proteolysis of oligodendrocyte proteins is associated with the activation of calpain-1 in the rhesus monkey. *J. Neurochem.* 2003, 84, 157-168.

Sternberger S, Poewe W, Wenning GK, Stefanova N. Targeted overexpression of human alpha-synuclein in oligodendroglia induces lesions linked to

MSA-like progressive autonomic failure. *Exp. Neurol.* 2010, 224, 459-464.

Storch M, Lassman H. Pathology and pathogenesis of demyelinating diseases. *Curr. Opin. Neurol.* 1997, 10, 186-192.

Syed A, Armstrong RA, Smith CUM. Quantification of axonal loss in Alzheimer's disease. *Alz. Rep.* 2000, 3, 19-24.

Tanaka J, Okuma Y, Tomobe K, Nomura Y. The age-related degeneration of oligodendrocytes in the hippocampus of the senescence-accelerated mouse (SAM) P8: a quantitative immunohistochemical study. *Biol. Pharm. Bull* 2005, 28, 615-618.

Thomas JL, Spassky N, Perez-Villegas EM, Olivier C, Cobos I, Goujet-Zalc C, Martinez S, Zalc B. Spatiotemporal development of oligodendrocytes in the embryonic brain. *J. Neurosci. Res.* 2000, 59, 471-476.

Tkachev D, Mimmack ML, Ryan MM et al., Oligodendrocyte dysfunction in schizophrenia and bipolar disorder. *Lancet* 2003, 362, 798-805.

Ubhi K, Rockenstein E, Mante M, Inglis C, Adame A, Patrick C, Whitney K, Masliah E. Neurodegeneration in a transgenic mouse model of multiple system atrophy is associated with altered expression of oligodendroglial-derived neurotrophic factors. *J. Neurosci.* 2010, 30, 6236-6246.

Wenning GK, Tison F, Ben-Shlomo Y, Daniel SE, Quinn NP. Multiple system atrophy: a review of 203 pathologically proven cases. *Move Disord.* 1997, 12, 133-147.

In: Oligodendrocytes
Editor: Dana Swanson
ISBN: 978-1-63483-330-1

Chapter 2

Microglia As Modulators of Oligodendrocyte Fate

Luisa Torres and Stella E. Tsirka
Program in Molecular and Cellular Pharmacology Stony Brook University, New York, Department of Pharmacological Sciences, Stony Brook University, NY, US

Abstract

Microglia have the potential for shaping the formation of new oligodendrocytes and controlling myelination and remyelination through direct and indirect mechanisms. Likewise, oligodendrocytes have functions that go beyond myelin production and extend to modulating microglial behavior and activation. Here, we review the effects of microglia on oligodendrocytes in both physiological and pathological conditions. We focus on the outcomes of the microglia-oligodendrocyte interaction in terms of myelination, oligodendrocyte differentiation, oligodendrocyte death, and remyelination while highlighting the influence of the activation state of microglia on the outcome of such interactions.

Introduction

Microglia are the first line of defense against disease in the central nervous system (CNS). They originate from $CD45^{-}$c-kit^{+} yolk-sac precursors that invade the brain using matrix metalloproteinases (MMPs), such as MMP-8 and MMP-9 (Kierdorf et al., 2013). These precursors eventually develop into $CD45^{+}$c-$kit^{-}$$CX3CR1^{+}$ microglia prior to the formation of the blood-brain barrier. During prenatal development microglia possess an ameboid shape and more closely resemble macrophages. Microglia then undergo proliferation and acquire ramified processes (Nayak et al., 2014). Once they fully colonize the brain parenchyma several factors including Colony Stimulating Factor -1 (Csf-1), Runx1, PU.1, Interferon Regulatory Factor 8 (IRF-8), and miR-124 contribute to their maintenance and self-renewal (Nayak et al., 2014; Wegiel et al., 1998).

Microglia play key roles in several neurological diseases and can quickly respond to infection or injury (Colton & Wilcock, 2010b; Kraft & Harry, 2011). Two-photon microscopy studies revealed that microglia use their processes to constantly survey the brain parenchyma in order to react to potential insults (Nimmerjahn et al., 2005). This perpetual surveying state allows microglia to serve important functions both under physiological and pathological conditions. In the healthy CNS, microglia phagocytose apoptotic cells, prune synapses, and support the formation of neural circuits (Paolicelli et al., 2011; Ueno et al., 2013). Under pathological conditions, microglia become activated and initiate an inflammatory response characterized by microglia proliferation, upregulation of a large number of microglial receptors, and cytokine production (Colton & Wilcock, 2010b; Hanisch, 2002; Kraft & Harry, 2011). Activated microglia may be classified into at least two categories: M1 or pro-inflammatory microglia are characterized by production of tumor necrosis factor -α (TNFα), interleukin 1β (IL-1β), and IL-6 (Colton & Wilcock, 2010a; Varnum & Ikezu, 2012) ; and M2 or anti-inflammatory microglia are characterized by production of IL-10, transforming growth factor-β (TGFβ), IL-4, and IL-14. M2 microglia are considered beneficial for regeneration and repair in several CNS disorders, while M1 microglia favor continued inflammation and tissue injury (Kigerl et al., 2009; Miron et al., 2013).

Besides their roles in mediating the inflammatory response, microglia also play an important supportive role in the CNS (Nayak et al., 2014; Paolicelli et al., 2011; Schwartz et al., 2013). During early neurogenesis microglia phagocytose apoptotic cells, eliminate unwanted neuronal projections, and control production of cortical neurons by regulating the proliferation and survival of neural precursor cells (Aarum et al., 2003; Cunningham, 2013; Deierborg et al., 2010; Guadagno et al., 2013; Monje et al., 2003; Paolicelli et al., 2011; Schafer et al., 2012; Sierra et al., 2010). Microglia also provide trophic support for the formation of neuronal circuits and may be found adjacent to clusters of $PDGF^+$ oligodendrocyte progenitors during the development of cerebral white matter tracts, indicating a role for microglia in developmental processes such as neurogenesis, myelination, and oligodendrocyte formation (Ellison & de Vellis, 1995; Hamilton & Rome, 1994; Ueno et al., 2013).

Oligodendrocytes develop from progenitors known as oligodendrocyte precursor cells (OPCs), which proliferate in the sub-ventricular zone (SVZ) and migrate towards various zones in the brain where they become mature cells (Baumann & Pham-Dinh, 2001; Miller, 2002; Noble, 2000). This sequence of events occurs both during development and in demyelinating conditions (Baumann & Pham-Dinh, 2001; McTigue et al., 1998; Woodruff et al., 2004). During the differentiation process, OPCs downregulate expression of neuron-glial antigen 2 (NG2) and alpha-type platelet-derived growth factor receptor (PDGFRα), and upregulate expression of 2',3'-Cyclic-nucleotide 3'-phosphodiesterase (CNPase), adenomatous polyposis coli (APC), and myelin basic protein (MBP) (McTigue & Tripathi, 2008). Differentiation requires the action of several transcription factors known to interact with the promoters of myelin-specific genes. These include Olig1, Olig2, Nkx2.2, Nkx2.6, MyT1, and sex determining region Y box (Sox)-10 (Miron et al., 2011). Mature oligodendrocytes ensure rapid transmission of electrical impulses by forming protective myelin sheaths around axons(McTigue & Tripathi, 2008). Besides being responsible for myelin production, oligodendrocytes maintain axonal integrity and support axonal metabolism and neuronal survival (Funfschilling et al., 2012). If oligodendrocytes become damaged, motor, sensory, and cognitive deficits may occur. Although myelination occurs early in life OPCs retain their capacity to differentiate into mature oligodendrocytes and migrate to sites of demyelination during adulthood. Experimental OPC ablation or differentiation results in the rapid mobilization of OPCs to replace dead or differentiated progenitors, thus ensuring that their density is maintained (Hughes et al., 2013).

Oligodendrocytes and their precursors are particularly vulnerable to apoptotic cell death during CNS injury. Their high amounts of intracellular iron and relatively low levels of antioxidant enzymes makes them highly vulnerable to oxidative stress (Thorburne & Juurlink, 1996). Multiple pathologies, including Alzheimer's disease, spinal cord injury, Parkinson's disease, ischemia, and hypoxia are characterized by oligodendrocyte loss along with microglial activation (Chew et al., 2013; Deng et al., 2008; Domercq et al., 2010; Merrill & Scolding, 1999; Peferoen et al., 2014; Varnum & Ikezu, 2012). Here, we review recent advances on understanding the effects of microglia on oligodendrocyte biology, including the effects of microglia on oligodendrocyte formation, cell death, myelination, and remyelination. Better understanding of the dialogue between microglia and oligodendrocytes is critical for understanding the progression of various CNS disorders and for identifying new targets to aid the repair process.

Microglia in Oligogenesis and Myelination

Early studies on the effect of microglia on myelination found that levels of myelin-specific proteins and galactolipids such as sulfatide, MBP, and, proteolipid protein (PLP) increase when microglia are co-cultured with oligodendrocytes (Hamilton & Rome, 1994). Microglial-conditioned media accelerates the differentiation of cultured oligodendrocytes, indicating that cell-to-cell contact is not necessary for differentiation to occur (Hamilton & Rome, 1994; Pang et al., 2013). In co-cultures of neurons and oligodendrocytes, microglial-conditioned media strongly promotes myelination(Pang et al., 2013). Microglia may also regulate myelin thickness and compaction, as Galectin-3, a protein abundant in phagocytic microglia, promotes oligodendrocyte formation and plays a role in maintaining myelin integrity (Pasquini et al., 2011; Reichert & Rotshenker, 1999).

Soluble factors released by microglia have an effect on OPC survival and oligodendrocyte formation (Almad et al., 2011; Palazuelos et al., 2014; Tripathi & McTigue, 2007) (Table 1). A detailed look at microglia morphology and distribution in the neonatal rat forebrain revealed a cytokine-dependent role for microglia in oligogenesis. Ameboid microglia massively accumulate in the SVZ during the first ten days following birth, reaching a peak at P4 (Goings et al., 2006; Marshall et al., 2008; Shigemoto-Mogami et al., 2014). High mRNA levels of both pro-inflammatory and anti-inflammatory cytokines are observed during this developmental period (Crain et al., 2013). Minocycline administration from P2 to P4 results in a decrease in pro-inflammatory cytokines along with reduced numbers of MBP^+ cells and more PDGF+ OPCs, indicating an effect of activated microglia and the cytokines they release on oligodendrocyte differentiation.

Table 1. Soluble factors released by microglia affect OPCs and oligodendrocytes

List of the most common microglia-derived cytokines and soluble factors along with their known effects on OPCs and oligodendrocytes

	Cytokine	Effect on OPCs	Effect on oligodedrocytes	Reference
M1	IFN-γ	Differentiation ↓ Proliferation ↑	Cell death ↑	(Buntinx et al., 2004b) (Lin et al., 2006)
	IL-1β	Proliferation ↑ Differentiation ↑	Cell death ↑	(Miron et al., 2011; Pang et al., 2003)
	TNFα	Proliferation ↑ Differentiation ↓	Cell death ↑	(Arnett et al., 2001) (Bonora et al., 2014; Nakazawa et al., 2006)
	IL-6	Proliferation ↑ Differentiation ↑	Cell death ↓	(Zhang et al., 2004)
M2	IL-10	Unknown	Cell death ↓	(Molina-Holgado et al., 2001)
	IL-4	Differentiation ↑	Cell death ↓	(Molina-Holgado et al., 2001)
	CNTF	Proliferation ↑ Differentiation ↑	Cell death ↓	(Talbott et al., 2007)
	IGF-1	Proliferation ↑ Differentiation ↑	Cell death ↓	(Mason et al., 2003) (Nicholas et al., 2002; Pang et al., 2007)
	TGFβ	Migration ↑ Differentiation ↑	Cell death ↓	(Lalive et al., 2005; McKinnon et al., 1993)
	IL-11	Proliferation ↑ Differentiation ↑	Cell death ↓	(Zhang et al., 2006)

In vivo models of demyelination have shown that anti-inflammatory cytokines favor oligogenesis. Microglia switch from M1 to M2 during the remyelination phase after lysolecithin injection (Miron et al., 2013). This switch occurs along with expression of Activin-A. In vivo depletion of M2 microglia reduces the expression of MBP and Myelin Oligodendrocyte Glycoprotein (MOG) and reduces the number of nodes of Ranvier ten days after lysolecithin injection (Miron et al., 2013). In vitro experiments using oligodendrocytes treated with conditioned media derived from M1 or M2 polarized microglia showed that only the conditioned media from M2 microglia prevents apoptosis in serum and growth factor deprived OPCs. Similarly, only M2 conditioned media increases OPC differentiation into myelinating oligodendrocytes, indicating a role for M2 microglia in oligodendrocyte differentiation and suggesting that direct contact between oligodendrocytes and microglia is not necessary for oligogenesis to occur (Figure 1) (Hamilton & Rome, 1994; Miron et al., 2013).

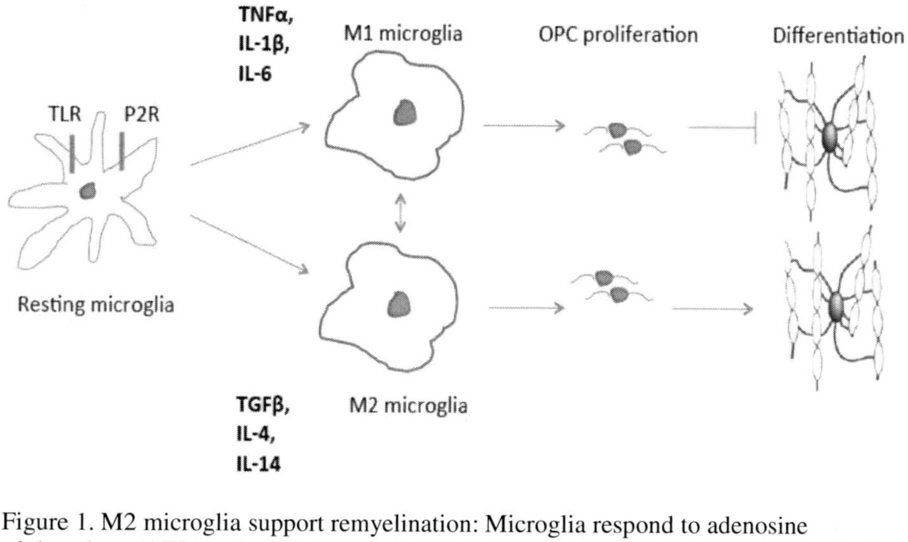

Figure 1. M2 microglia support remyelination: Microglia respond to adenosine triphosphate (ATP) and other extracellular ions within minutes after CNS injury via P2 receptors (P2R). Microglia exist in a continuum between two extreme states: The M1 or pro-inflammatory state characterized by production of TNFα, IL-1β, and IL-6, and the anti-inflammatory M2 state characterized by production of IL-10, Transforming growth factor-β (TGFβ), IL-4, and IL-14. Although both M1 and M2 microglia/macrophages favor OPC proliferation, only M2 microglia are supportive of formation of myelinating oligodendrocytes.

Microglia activated with the anti-inflammatory cytokine IL-4 can induce the formation of new oligodendrocytes (Butovsky et al., 2006b), while activation with Interferon- γ (IFN-γ) impedes oligogenesis from neural precursor cells (NPCs) (Butovsky et al., 2006a). IL-4 reverses this impediment by inducing production of insulin growth factor -1 (IGF-1) and lowering TNF-α levels. In rats undergoing experimental autoimmune encephalomyelitis (EAE), treatment with IL-4 increases oligogenesis and improves clinical symptoms. (Butovsky et al., 2006a).

Although a lot of evidence points towards a direct effect of microglia on oligogenesis through the release of cytokines, they could also have indirect effects by inducing growth factor release from astrocytes. For instance, microglia/macrophage TNFα promotes production of neurotrophin and cilliary neurotrophic factor (CNTF) in astrocytes (Schonberg et al., 2007). Similarly, microglia/macrophage IL-1β induces astrocytic production of IGF-1, which is crucial for successful remyelination and oligodendrocyte survival (Talbott et al., 2005; Zeger et al., 2007). IL-1β and TGF-β induce astrocytic production of IL-11, which reduces oligodendrocyte apoptosis and favors myelination (Zhang et al., 2006). Activated microglia may also affect OPCs and oligodendrocytes indirectly by controlling the proliferation and survival of NPCs (Aarum et al., 2003; Cunningham, 2013; Deierborg et al., 2010; Guadagno et al., 2013; Monje et al., 2003).

Microglia-Derived Iron As a Pro-Oligogenic Signal

Iron accumulation is necessary for proper oligodendrocyte formation and myelination during development (Zecca et al., 2004). Lack of iron reduces microglia-produced TNF-α and IL-1β, both of which are involved in iron uptake and remyelination (Arnett et al., 2001; Rathore et al., 2012; Schulz et al., 2012). Microglia accumulate iron before the onset of myelination and then release it to OPCs before they become myelinating cells (Todorich et al., 2009). A few studies show that iron might act as a bridge for the effective communication between microglia and oligodendrocytes. For instance, microglia-derived ferritin is taken up by oligodendrocytes ultimately favoring OPC proliferation and oligodendrocyte survival (Hulet et al., 2000). Iron chelation by deferasirox after intraspinal Lipopolysaccharide (LPS) treatment abolishes ferritin expression in OPCs and oligodendrocytes, leading to a decrease in OPC proliferation and differentiation and supporting the role of ferritin as a pro-oligogenic signal (Almad et al., 2011; Schonberg & McTigue, 2009).

Although iron uptake is essential for myelination, extremely high levels of intracellular iron make oligodendrocytes vulnerable to oxidative stress (Thorburne & Juurlink, 1996). Primary oligodendrocytes treated with conditioned medium from hypoxic microglia exhibit reduced glutathione levels, increased lipid peroxidation, upregulated caspase-3 expression, and reduced proliferation (Rathnasamy et al., 2011). These effects are reversed upon treatment with conditioned medium from hypoxic microglia previously treated with iron chelator deferoxamine indicating that excess iron derived from microglia might mediate oligodendrocyte cell death.

Microglia in Oligodendrocyte Apoptosis

Oligodendrocytes express both AMPA and NMDA receptors which makes them vulnerable to glutamate-mediated apoptosis (Karadottir et al., 2005; McTigue & Tripathi, 2008). One major potential glutamate source is microglia (Domercq et al., 2007; Piani & Fontana, 1994). Elevated glutamate levels have been described in several CNS pathologies including stroke, amyotrophic lateral sclerosis, Parkinson's disease, and spinal cord injury (Davalos et al., 1997; Follett et al., 2004; Foran & Trotti, 2009; Johnson et al., 2009; Park et al., 2004).

Microglia accumulate in great numbers around demyelinated areas (Clarner et al., 2012; Remington et al., 2007) and are found in close contact with dying oligodendrocytes (Shuman et al., 1997). In addition, major myelin proteins, such as PLP, can be detected within Iba-1^{+} microglia/macrophages. Some studies have shown a direct effect of microglia on oligodendrocyte apoptosis through the release of reactive oxygen and reactive nitrogen species (Li et al., 2005; Merrill et al., 1993; Yeo et al., 2012). Although OPCs are especially susceptible to cytotoxic factors in culture (Husain & Juurlink, 1995; Thorburne & Juurlink, 1996), fully differentiated oligodendrocytes, although also vulnerable, seem to cope better with oxidative stress compared to OPCs(Kim et al., 2013). In microglia-oligodendrocyte co-cultures microglia can have detrimental or beneficial effects on oligodendrocytes depending on the activation state of microglia as well as the differentiation state of the oligodendrocytes (Nicholas et al., 2003). While inactive microglia protect OPCs (Nicholas et al., 2001), microglia and macrophages isolated from contused spinal cords inhibit OPC growth through the release of soluble factors (Wu et al., 2010). Similarly, whereas cultured activated microglia reduce OPC survival, microglia seem to have a protective effect on mature oligodendrocytes regardless of their activation state (Miller et al., 2007; Nicholas et al., 2002).

The effects of microglial activation on OPCs and oligodendrocytes may also depend on which Toll-like receptor is stimulated on microglia. The TLR2 agonist zymosan causes total axon and oligodendrocyte loss without formation of new oligodendrocytes, whereas treatment with the TLR4 agonist LPS causes acute oligodendrocyte loss followed by massive OPC proliferation and oligodendrocyte replacement(Schonberg et al., 2007; Skripuletz et al., 2011). LPS-induced neurotrophin-3 may account for the positive effects on new oligodendrocyte formation.

The duration of microglial stimulation has an effect on the outcome of the interaction between microglia and oligodendrocytes. 24-hour in-vitro stimulation of microglia with LPS markedly increases production of pro-inflammatory cytokines and reduces survival of NPCs, whereas chronic LPS stimulation reduces production of pro-inflammatory cytokines and favors anti-inflammatory factors along with NPC survival (Cacci et al., 2008).

Although microglial activation results in the release of factors that can be harmful to other cells (Buntinx et al., 2004a; Li et al., 2008; Pang et al., 2003), microglia can also release anti-inflammatory mediators that may offset the harmful impact of pro-inflammatory cytokines. For example, microglia-produced IGF-1 reduces oligodendrocyte death caused by high levels of TNFα (Nicholas et al., 2002). Similarly, IL-4 induces expression of IGF-1 and reverses the inhibition of oligogenesis caused by microglial activation with IFN-γ (Butovsky et al., 2006a).

Microglia in Demyelination and Remyelination

Demyelinating lesions occur in the CNS as a result of oligodendrocyte death following CNS trauma. Formation of new myelinating oligodendrocytes is required for remyelination to occur, as existing mature oligodendrocytes are post-mitotic and unable to migrate(Miron et al., 2011). In order to repair the damaged axons, OPCs must proliferate and migrate towards the demyelinating region (Baumann & Pham-Dinh, 2001; Miller, 2002; Noble, 2000). OPC activation requires the adoption of a hypertrophic morphology and an increase in responsiveness to mitogens and chemoattractants (Miron et al., 2011). M1 microglia play a crucial role in OPC recruitment (Miron et al., 2013). Microglia and macrophage- derived chemokines and cytokines such as TNFα, IL-1β, IL-11 and CXCL-2 increase OPC proliferation, migration, and differentiation (Miron et al., 2011). The phenotype of microglia may change depending on whether demyelination or remyelination is occurring. Microglia dramatically increase their phagocytic activity and expression of phagocytic receptors such as TREM-2b during demyelination. TNF-α is increased at this stage, while levels of IL-10 and TGF-β remain unchanged (Voss et al., 2012). This high production of TNF-α contributes to OPC recruitment to demyelinated areas (Arnett et al., 2001; Miron et al., 2013). However, a switch to the M2 phenotype is required to aid in the differentiation process from OPCs to myelinating oligodendrocytes (Miron et al., 2013) (Figure 1). In fact, brain areas in which active remyelination is occurring contain significantly higher numbers of M2 macrophages compared to areas in which there is no active remyelination (Boven et al., 2006). In contrast, a different study showed that the microglia phenotype during both demyelination and remyelination is remarkably similar and found no evidence for the existence of a microglia phenotype supportive of exclusively demyelination or remyelination (Olah et al., 2012). Microarray analyses revealed that genes associated with myelin phagocytosis, recycling of myelin components, tissue remodeling, OPC recruitment, and trophic support for OPCs and oligodendrocytes were highly upregulated during both demyelination and remyelination (Olah et al., 2012). Genes associated with major histocompatibility complex II such as CD74, H2-Aa, and H2-Ab1 are also highly upregulated during both stages. Similarly, microglia upregulate M1-type markers such as TLR4, Lyz1 and Lyz2, TNF-α, IL-1β, and MMP-12 and M2-specific markers such as IL-13, IL-4 during both demyelination and remyelination(Olah et al., 2012). This latter study did not compare M1 gene expression relative to M2 gene expression. Therefore, it is possible that gene expression characteristic of both M1 and M2 microglia/macrophes is present during both demyelination and remyelination. However, signals from the microenvieronment allow cytokines derived from M1 type microglia to predominate during demyelination, while cytokynes derived from M2 microglia/macrophages offset the effects of M1 derived cytokines during remyelination. Future work should focus on characterizing whether microglia exist as distinct populations of M1 and M2 cells, or whether the same cells can reverse their phenotype depending on the signals they receive.

It was recently shown that $NG2^+$ OPCs take 48 hours to differentiate into APC^+ oligodendrocytes during postnatal development, providing ample time for cues in the microenvironment to control oligodendrocyte differentiation (Hill et al., 2014). Newly generated oligodendrocytes form around lesions and are surrounded by microglia and macrophages (Mabuchi et al., 2000; Mandai et al., 1997). Similarly, upregulation of PLP mRNA occurs concomitantly with macrophage infiltration in a model of spinal cord injury (Frei et al., 2000). Several studies indicate that remyelination cannot occur in the absence of microglia/macrophages (Imai et al., 2008; Kotter et al., 2001; Lampron et al., 2015), as they remove myelin debris which contains potent inhibitors of OPC differentiation, release trophic factors that promote neuronal regeneration, and recycle cholesterol and other myelin lipids to use as trophic support to remyelinating oligodendroctyes (Olah et al., 2012; Rabchevsky & Streit, 1997). For instance, demyelination is equally severe in both wild-type and CX3CR1-deficient mice after cuprizone treatment. However, the clearance of myelin debris in mice lacking CX3CR1 is severely impaired resulting in loss of axon integrity and incomplete remyelination (Lampron et al., 2015), indicating that without myelin clearance proper remyelination cannot occur. Microglia and macrophages persist for months in both spinal cord injuries and multiple sclerotic lesions (Hausmann, 2003; Prineas et al., 2001) and continue to release cytokines, chemokines, and growth factors (Gao & Tsirka, 2011). In the chronic phase of SCI microglia have regenerative effects, as grafting cultured microglia into injured spinal cord promotes axonal regrowth into the lesioned area (Rabchevsky & Streit, 1997). These effects may be due to the release of trophic factors such as nerve growth factor (NGF), neurotrophin-3 (NT-3), IL-1a, IL-10, brain derived growth factor (BDNF), and IGF-1. The latter has been shown to be necessary for remyelination as specific deletion of IGF-1 in the brain results in reduced OPC migration, proliferation, and survival (Mason et al., 2003).

Although microglia control oligodendrocyte fate through cytokine release, oligodendrocytes and their precursors play an active role in modulating microglia behavior and activation. For instance, NPCs have been found to regulate microglial proliferation, chemotaxis, and phagocytosis(Mosher et al., 2012). Specific deletion of β-catenin to reduce OPC proliferation after spinal cord injury reduces microglial activation (Rodriguez et al., 2014). Oligodendrocytes can release microglial chemokines in order to recruit microglia in moments of distress (Nicholas et al., 2003). Similarly, $NG2^+$ OPCs counteract the detrimental effect of microglia/macrophages on injured axons and provide a favorable substrate for axonal re-growth (Busch et al., 2010), indicating that oligodendrocytes and OPCs themselves have the potential to shape microglial fate and behavior.

Therapeutic Approaches to Reduce Microglial Activation and Improve Remyelination

The injured spinal cord and the multiple sclerosis brain are rich in molecules that are inhibitory for repair (Lau et al., 2012; Rolls et al., 2009). Examples of such molecules include Chondroitin Sulfate Proteoglycans (CSPGs) which form the glial scar and whose deposition is associated with reduced axonal re-growth (Davies et al., 1997; McKeon et al., 1991; Niederost et al., 1999; Smith-Thomas et al., 1994). In culture, CSPGs interfere with the adhesion, differentiation, and myelin production of human and mouse OPCs (Lau et al., 2012). Enzymatic degradation of CSPGs using Chondroitinase reverses these effects and increases OPC migration, axonal sprouting, and remyelination in a model of spinal cord injury and in mice demyelinated with lysolecithin (Lau et al., 2012; Siebert & Osterhout, 2011; Siebert et al., 2011). These effects are accompanied by functional improvements (Kanno et al., 2014; Wang et al., 2011). Chondroitinase can also induce an anti-inflammatory, phagocytic phenotype in microglia, supporting a role for the M2 state in oligogenesis and remyelination (Bartus et al., 2014; Ebert et al., 2008; Rolls et al., 2008).

A number of anti-inflammatory drugs have been used in animal studies to reduce microglial activation and improve disease outcome. Our lab has shown that targeting microglial function during the secondary phase of spinal cord injury ameliorates the injury outcome by improving oligodendrocyte differentiation and remyelination (Bukhari et al., 2011; Emmetsberger & Tsirka, 2012). Treatment with MIF/TKP inhibits microglial activation, enhances the proliferation of purified $NG2^{+}$ OPCs, and reduces oligodendrocyte apoptosis in a hemisection model of spinal cord injury (Emmetsberger & Tsirka, 2012). Transplantation of OPCs into the spinal cord of Long Evans shaker, a myelin mutant characterized by progressive microglia activation, results in failure of OPCs to survive and myelinate if transplanted during the peak of microglial activation. In contrast, pretreatment with Minocycline directly onto the spinal cord allows OPCs to survive, engraft, and myelinate successfully (Zhang et al., 2003). Minocycline has also been shown to inhibit the polarization of microglia towards the M1 state (Kobayashi et al., 2013) and has been shown to reduce oligodendrocyte death through inhibition of microglia-derived ProNGF (Yune et al., 2007).

Conclusion and Future Research

It is clear that microglia/ macrophages have considerable potential for shaping OPC responses both in the healthy CNS and during injury. The outcomes of the cross-talk between microglia and oligodendrocytes highly depend on the differentiation state of the oligodendrocytes, the activation state of microglia, the microglial receptors involved, and the duration of microglial activation. Understanding these differences is crucial to understanding developmental processes such as myelination, as well as the progression of diseases that involve chronic activation of microglia together with oligodendrocyte loss.

Future work should focus on extending the duration of the anti-inflammatory phenotype of microglia in order to overcome the remyelination failure characteristics of CNS disorders suchas multiple sclerosis. Microglia polarization and the ratio of M1:M2 microglia has only been examined through day 28 in a model of spinal cord injury and up to day 14 in a model of brain ischemia (Hu et al., 2012; Kigerl et al., 2009). Both studies coincide in that expression of anti-inflammatory factors is transient, while the M1 state predominates (Kigerl et al., 2009). However, the role of microglia and their activation state at more chronic time points is unknown. This would be important to determine in light of a study showing that the number of demyelinated axons increases progressively during a period of 450 days after spinal cord injury(Totoiu & Keirstead, 2005). This same study showed that ongoing remyelination at chronic time points post injury is incomplete and inefficient as unmyelinated axons are observed throughout the 450 day period.

In vitro studies looking at the interplay between microglia and oligodendrocytes should include human microglia as it is unknown whether they respond in a similar way compared to rodent microglia. For example, while mouse microglia highly express the LPS receptor Toll-like receptor 4, human microglia have low levels of expression of this receptor (Melief et al., 2012; Smith & Dragunow, 2014), which would undermine the numerous studies that have been conducted examining the effect of LPS-activated microglia on OPC survival and differentiation.

Acknowledgments

We thank the members of the Tsirka and Colognato labs for helpful discussions. This work was supported by NIH R01NS42168 and TRO Fusion Award from Stony Brook School of Medicine and the Office of the Vice President for Research (SET), and Turner Dissertation funds to LT.

References

Aarum J, Sandberg K, Haeberlein SL, Persson MA (2003) Migration and differentiation of neural precursor cells can be directed by microglia. *Proc Natl Acad Sci U S A* 100: 15983-15988.

Almad A, Sahinkaya FR, McTigue DM (2011) Oligodendrocyte fate after spinal cord injury. *Neurotherapeutics* 8: 262-273.

Arnett HA, Mason J, Marino M, Suzuki K, Matsushima GK, Ting JP (2001) TNF alpha promotes proliferation of oligodendrocyte progenitors and remyelination. *Nat Neurosci* 4: 1116-1122.

Bartus K, James ND, Didangelos A, Bosch KD, Verhaagen J, Yanez-Munoz RJ, Rogers JH, Schneider BL, Muir EM, Bradbury EJ (2014) Large-scale chondroitin sulfate proteoglycan digestion with chondroitinase gene therapy leads to reduced pathology and modulates macrophage phenotype following spinal cord contusion injury. *J Neurosci* 34: 4822-4836.

Baumann N, Pham-Dinh D (2001) Biology of oligodendrocyte and myelin in the mammalian central nervous system. *Physiol Rev* 81: 871-927.

Bonora M, De Marchi E, Patergnani S, Suski JM, Celsi F, Bononi A, Giorgi C, Marchi S, Rimessi A, Duszynski J, Pozzan T, Wieckowski MR, Pinton P (2014) Tumor necrosis factor-alpha impairs oligodendroglial differentiation through a mitochondria-dependent process. *Cell Death Differ* 21: 1198-1208.

Boven LA, Van Meurs M, Van Zwam M, Wierenga-Wolf A, Hintzen RQ, Boot RG, Aerts JM, Amor S, Nieuwenhuis EE, Laman JD (2006) Myelin-laden macrophages are anti-inflammatory, consistent with foam cells in multiple sclerosis. *Brain* 129: 517-526.

Bukhari N, Torres L, Robinson JK, Tsirka SE (2011) Axonal Regrowth after Spinal Cord Injury via Chondroitinase and the Tissue Plasminogen Activator (tPA)/Plasmin System. *J Neurosci* 31: 14931-14943.

Buntinx M, Gielen E, Van Hummelen P, Raus J, Ameloot M, Steels P, Stinissen P (2004a) Cytokine-induced cell death in human oligodendroglial cell lines. II: Alterations in gene expression induced by interferon-gamma and tumor necrosis factor-alpha. *J Neurosci Res* 76: 846-861.

Buntinx M, Moreels M, Vandenabeele F, Lambrichts I, Raus J, Steels P, Stinissen P, Ameloot M (2004b) Cytokine-induced cell death in human oligodendroglial cell lines: I. Synergistic effects of IFN-gamma and TNF-alpha on apoptosis. *J Neurosci Res* 76: 834-845.

Busch SA, Horn KP, Cuascut FX, Hawthorne AL, Bai L, Miller RH, Silver J (2010) Adult NG2+ cells are permissive to neurite outgrowth and stabilize sensory axons during macrophage-induced axonal dieback after spinal cord injury. *J Neurosci* 30: 255-265.

Butovsky O, Landa G, Kunis G, Ziv Y, Avidan H, Greenberg N, Schwartz A, Smirnov I, Pollack A, Jung S, Schwartz M (2006a) Induction and blockage of oligodendrogenesis by differently activated microglia in an animal model of multiple sclerosis. *J Clin Invest* 116: 905-915.

Butovsky O, Ziv Y, Schwartz A, Landa G, Talpalar AE, Pluchino S, Martino G, Schwartz M (2006b) Microglia activated by IL-4 or IFN-gamma differentially induce neurogenesis and oligodendrogenesis from adult stem/progenitor cells. *Mol Cell Neurosci* 31: 149-160.

Cacci E, Ajmone-Cat MA, Anelli T, Biagioni S, Minghetti L (2008) In vitro neuronal and glial differentiation from embryonic or adult neural precursor cells are differently affected by chronic or acute activation of microglia. *Glia* 56: 412-425.

Chew LJ, Fusar-Poli P, Schmitz T (2013) Oligodendroglial alterations and the role of microglia in white matter injury: relevance to schizophrenia. *Dev Neurosci* 35: 102-129.

Clarner T, Diederichs F, Berger K, Denecke B, Gan L, van der Valk P, Beyer C, Amor S, Kipp M (2012) Myelin debris regulates inflammatory responses in an experimental demyelination animal model and multiple sclerosis lesions. *Glia* 60: 1468-1480.

Colton C, Wilcock DM (2010a) Assessing activation states in microglia. *CNS Neurol Disord Drug Targets* 9: 174-191.

Colton CA, Wilcock DM (2010b) Assessing activation states in microglia. *CNS Neurol Disord Drug Targets* 9: 174-191.

Crain JM, Nikodemova M, Watters JJ (2013) Microglia express distinct M1 and M2 phenotypic markers in the postnatal and adult central nervous system in male and female mice. *J Neurosci Res* 91: 1143-1151.

Cunningham C (2013) Microglia and neurodegeneration: the role of systemic inflammation. *Glia* 61: 71-90.

Davalos A, Castillo J, Serena J, Noya M (1997) Duration of glutamate release after acute ischemic stroke. *Stroke* 28: 708-710.

Davies SJ, Fitch MT, Memberg SP, Hall AK, Raisman G, Silver J (1997) Regeneration of adult axons in white matter tracts of the central nervous system. *Nature* 390: 680-683.

Deierborg T, Roybon L, Inacio AR, Pesic J, Brundin P (2010) Brain injury activates microglia that induce neural stem cell proliferation ex vivo and promote differentiation of neurosphere-derived cells into neurons and oligodendrocytes. *Neuroscience* 171: 1386-1396.

Deng Y, Lu J, Sivakumar V, Ling EA, Kaur C (2008) Amoeboid microglia in the periventricular white matter induce oligodendrocyte damage through expression of proinflammatory cytokines via MAP kinase signaling pathway in hypoxic neonatal rats. *Brain Pathol* 18: 387-400.

Domercq M, Perez-Samartin A, Aparicio D, Alberdi E, Pampliega O, Matute C (2010) P2X7 receptors mediate ischemic damage to oligodendrocytes. *Glia* 58: 730-740.

Domercq M, Sanchez-Gomez MV, Sherwin C, Etxebarria E, Fern R, Matute C (2007) System xc- and glutamate transporter inhibition mediates microglial toxicity to oligodendrocytes. *J Immunol* 178: 6549-6556.

Ebert S, Schoeberl T, Walczak Y, Stoecker K, Stempfl T, Moehle C, Weber BH, Langmann T (2008) Chondroitin sulfate disaccharide stimulates microglia to adopt a novel regulatory phenotype. *J Leukoc Biol* 84: 736-740.

Ellison JA, de Vellis J (1995) Amoeboid microglia expressing GD3 ganglioside are concentrated in regions of oligodendrogenesis during development of the rat corpus callosum. *Glia* 14: 123-132.

Emmetsberger J, Tsirka SE (2012) Microglial inhibitory factor (MIF/TKP) mitigates secondary damage following spinal cord injury. *Neurobiol Dis* 47: 295-309.

Follett PL, Deng W, Dai W, Talos DM, Massillon LJ, Rosenberg PA, Volpe JJ, Jensen FE (2004) Glutamate receptor-mediated oligodendrocyte toxicity in periventricular leukomalacia: a protective role for topiramate. *J Neurosci* 24: 4412-4420.

Foran E, Trotti D (2009) Glutamate transporters and the excitotoxic path to motor neuron degeneration in amyotrophic lateral sclerosis. *Antioxid Redox Signal* 11: 1587-1602.

Frei E, Klusman I, Schnell L, Schwab ME (2000) Reactions of oligodendrocytes to spinal cord injury: cell survival and myelin repair. *Exp Neurol* 163: 373-380.

Funfschilling U, Supplie LM, Mahad D, Boretius S, Saab AS, Edgar J, Brinkmann BG, Kassmann CM, Tzvetanova ID, Mobius W, Diaz F, Meijer D, Suter U, Hamprecht B, Sereda MW, Moraes CT, Frahm J, Goebbels S, Nave KA (2012) Glycolytic oligodendrocytes maintain myelin and long-term axonal integrity. *Nature* 485: 517-521.

Gao Z, Tsirka SE (2011) Animal Models of MS Reveal Multiple Roles of Microglia in Disease Pathogenesis. *Neurol Res Int* 2011: 383087.

Goings GE, Kozlowski DA, Szele FG (2006) Differential activation of microglia in neurogenic versus non-neurogenic regions of the forebrain. *Glia* 54: 329-342.

Guadagno J, Xu X, Karajgikar M, Brown A, Cregan SP (2013) Microglia-derived TNFalpha induces apoptosis in neural precursor cells via transcriptional activation of the Bcl-2 family member Puma. *Cell Death Dis* 4: e538.

Hamilton SP, Rome LH (1994) Stimulation of in vitro myelin synthesis by microglia. *Glia* 11: 326-335.

Hanisch UK (2002) Microglia as a source and target of cytokines. *Glia* 40: 140-155.

Hausmann ON (2003) Post-traumatic inflammation following spinal cord injury. *Spinal Cord* 41: 369-378.

Hill RA, Patel KD, Goncalves CM, Grutzendler J, Nishiyama A (2014) Modulation of oligodendrocyte generation during a critical temporal window after NG2 cell division. *Nat Neurosci* 17: 1518-1527.

Hu X, Li P, Guo Y, Wang H, Leak RK, Chen S, Gao Y, Chen J (2012) Microglia/macrophage polarization dynamics reveal novel mechanism of injury expansion after focal cerebral ischemia. *Stroke* 43: 3063-3070.

Hughes EG, Kang SH, Fukaya M, Bergles DE (2013) Oligodendrocyte progenitors balance growth with self-repulsion to achieve homeostasis in the adult brain. *Nat Neurosci* 16: 668-676.

Hulet SW, Heyliger SO, Powers S, Connor JR (2000) Oligodendrocyte progenitor cells internalize ferritin via clathrin-dependent receptor mediated endocytosis. *J Neurosci Res* 61: 52-60.

Husain J, Juurlink BH (1995) Oligodendroglial precursor cell susceptibility to hypoxia is related to poor ability to cope with reactive oxygen species. *Brain Res* 698: 86-94.

Imai M, Watanabe M, Suyama K, Osada T, Sakai D, Kawada H, Matsumae M, Mochida J (2008) Delayed accumulation of activated macrophages and inhibition of remyelination after spinal cord injury in an adult rodent model. *J Neurosurg Spine* 8: 58-66.

Johnson KA, Conn PJ, Niswender CM (2009) Glutamate receptors as therapeutic targets for Parkinson's disease. *CNS Neurol Disord Drug Targets* 8: 475-491.

Kanno H, Pressman Y, Moody A, Berg R, Muir EM, Rogers JH, Ozawa H, Itoi E, Pearse DD, Bunge MB (2014) Combination of engineered Schwann cell grafts to secrete neurotrophin and chondroitinase promotes axonal regeneration and locomotion after spinal cord injury. *J Neurosci* 34: 1838-1855.

Karadottir R, Cavelier P, Bergersen LH, Attwell D (2005) NMDA receptors are expressed in oligodendrocytes and activated in ischaemia. *Nature* 438: 1162-1166.

Kierdorf K, Erny D, Goldmann T, Sander V, Schulz C, Perdiguero EG, Wieghofer P, Heinrich A, Riemke P, Holscher C, Muller DN, Luckow B, Brocker T, Debowski K, Fritz G, Opdenakker G, Diefenbach A, Biber K, Heikenwalder M, Geissmann F, Rosenbauer F, Prinz M (2013) Microglia emerge from erythromyeloid precursors via Pu.1- and Irf8-dependent pathways. *Nat Neurosci* 16: 273-280.

Kigerl KA, Gensel JC, Ankeny DP, Alexander JK, Donnelly DJ, Popovich PG (2009) Identification of two distinct macrophage subsets with divergent effects causing either neurotoxicity or regeneration in the injured mouse spinal cord. *J Neurosci* 29: 13435-13444.

Kim JY, Lee EY, Sohn HJ, Kim SW, Kim CH, Ahn HY, Kim DW, Cho SS, Seo JH (2013) Differential expression of alphaB-crystallin causes maturation-dependent susceptibility of oligodendrocytes to oxidative stress. *BMB Rep* 46: 501-506.

Kobayashi K, Imagama S, Ohgomori T, Hirano K, Uchimura K, Sakamoto K, Hirakawa A, Takeuchi H, Suzumura A, Ishiguro N, Kadomatsu K (2013) Minocycline selectively inhibits M1 polarization of microglia. *Cell Death Dis* 4: e525.

Kotter MR, Setzu A, Sim FJ, Van Rooijen N, Franklin RJ (2001) Macrophage depletion impairs oligodendrocyte remyelination following lysolecithin-induced demyelination. *Glia* 35: 204-212.

Kraft AD, Harry GJ (2011) Features of microglia and neuroinflammation relevant to environmental exposure and neurotoxicity. *Int J Environ Res Public Health* 8: 2980-3018.

Lalive PH, Paglinawan R, Biollaz G, Kappos EA, Leone DP, Malipiero U, Relvas JB, Moransard M, Suter T, Fontana A (2005) TGF-beta-treated microglia induce oligodendrocyte precursor cell chemotaxis through the HGF-c-Met pathway. *Eur J Immunol* 35: 727-737.

Lampron A, Larochelle A, Laflamme N, Prefontaine P, Plante MM, Sanchez MG, Yong VW, Stys PK, Tremblay ME, Rivest S (2015) Inefficient clearance of myelin debris by microglia impairs remyelinating processes. *J Exp Med.*

Lau LW, Keough MB, Haylock-Jacobs S, Cua R, Doring A, Sloka S, Stirling DP, Rivest S, Yong VW (2012) Chondroitin sulfate proteoglycans in demyelinated lesions impair remyelination. *Ann Neurol* 72: 419-432.

Li J, Baud O, Vartanian T, Volpe JJ, Rosenberg PA (2005) Peroxynitrite generated by inducible nitric oxide synthase and NADPH oxidase mediates microglial toxicity to oligodendrocytes. *Proc Natl Acad Sci U S A* 102: 9936-9941.

Li J, Ramenaden ER, Peng J, Koito H, Volpe JJ, Rosenberg PA (2008) Tumor necrosis factor alpha mediates lipopolysaccharide-induced microglial toxicity to developing oligodendrocytes when astrocytes are present. *J Neurosci* 28: 5321-5330.

Lin W, Kemper A, Dupree JL, Harding HP, Ron D, Popko B (2006) Interferon-gamma inhibits central nervous system remyelination through a process modulated by endoplasmic reticulum stress. *Brain* 129: 1306-1318.

Mabuchi T, Kitagawa K, Ohtsuki T, Kuwabara K, Yagita Y, Yanagihara T, Hori M, Matsumoto M (2000) Contribution of microglia/macrophages to expansion of infarction and response of oligodendrocytes after focal cerebral ischemia in rats. *Stroke* 31: 1735-1743.

Mandai K, Matsumoto M, Kitagawa K, Matsushita K, Ohtsuki T, Mabuchi T, Colman DR, Kamada T, Yanagihara T (1997) Ischemic damage and subsequent proliferation of oligodendrocytes in focal cerebral ischemia. *Neuroscience* 77: 849-861.

Marshall GP, 2nd, Demir M, Steindler DA, Laywell ED (2008) Subventricular zone microglia possess a unique capacity for massive in vitro expansion. *Glia* 56: 1799-1808.

Mason JL, Xuan S, Dragatsis I, Efstratiadis A, Goldman JE (2003) Insulin-like growth factor (IGF) signaling through type 1 IGF receptor plays an important role in remyelination. *J Neurosci* 23: 7710-7718.

McKeon RJ, Schreiber RC, Rudge JS, Silver J (1991) Reduction of neurite outgrowth in a model of glial scarring following CNS injury is correlated with the expression of inhibitory molecules on reactive astrocytes. *J Neurosci* 11: 3398-3411.

McKinnon RD, Piras G, Ida JA, Jr., Dubois-Dalcq M (1993) A role for TGF-beta in oligodendrocyte differentiation. *J Cell Biol* 121: 1397-1407.

McTigue DM, Horner PJ, Stokes BT, Gage FH (1998) Neurotrophin-3 and brain-derived neurotrophic factor induce oligodendrocyte proliferation and myelination of regenerating axons in the contused adult rat spinal cord. *J Neurosci* 18: 5354-5365.

McTigue DM, Tripathi RB (2008) The life, death, and replacement of oligodendrocytes in the adult CNS. *J Neurochem* 107: 1-19.

Melief J, Koning N, Schuurman KG, Van De Garde MD, Smolders J, Hoek RM, Van Eijk M, Hamann J, Huitinga I (2012) Phenotyping primary human microglia: tight regulation of LPS responsiveness. *Glia* 60: 1506-1517.

Merrill JE, Ignarro LJ, Sherman MP, Melinek J, Lane TE (1993) Microglial cell cytotoxicity of oligodendrocytes is mediated through nitric oxide. *J Immunol* 151: 2132-2141.

Merrill JE, Scolding NJ (1999) Mechanisms of damage to myelin and oligodendrocytes and their relevance to disease. *Neuropathol Appl Neurobiol* 25: 435-458.

Miller BA, Crum JM, Tovar CA, Ferguson AR, Bresnahan JC, Beattie MS (2007) Developmental stage of oligodendrocytes determines their response to activated microglia in vitro. *J Neuroinflammation* 4: 28.

Miller RH (2002) Regulation of oligodendrocyte development in the vertebrate CNS. *Prog Neurobiol* 67: 451-467.

Miron VE, Boyd A, Zhao JW, Yuen TJ, Ruckh JM, Shadrach JL, van Wijngaarden P, Wagers AJ, Williams A, Franklin RJ, ffrench-Constant C (2013) M2 microglia and macrophages drive oligodendrocyte differentiation during CNS remyelination. *Nat Neurosci* 16: 1211-1218.

Miron VE, Kuhlmann T, Antel JP (2011) Cells of the oligodendroglial lineage, myelination, and remyelination. *Biochim Biophys Acta* 1812: 184-193.

Molina-Holgado E, Vela JM, Arevalo-Martin A, Guaza C (2001) LPS/IFN-gamma cytotoxicity in oligodendroglial cells: role of nitric oxide and protection by the anti-inflammatory cytokine IL-10. *Eur J Neurosci* 13: 493-502.

Monje ML, Toda H, Palmer TD (2003) Inflammatory blockade restores adult hippocampal neurogenesis. *Science* 302: 1760-1765.

Mosher KI, Andres RH, Fukuhara T, Bieri G, Hasegawa-Moriyama M, He Y, Guzman R, Wyss-Coray T (2012) Neural progenitor cells regulate microglia functions and activity. *Nat Neurosci* 15: 1485-1487.

Nakazawa T, Nakazawa C, Matsubara A, Noda K, Hisatomi T, She H, Michaud N, Hafezi-Moghadam A, Miller JW, Benowitz LI (2006) Tumor necrosis factor-alpha mediates oligodendrocyte death and delayed retinal ganglion cell loss in a mouse model of glaucoma. *J Neurosci* 26: 12633-12641

Nayak D, Roth TL, McGavern DB (2014) Microglia development and function. *Annu Rev Immunol* 32: 367-402.

Nicholas R, Stevens S, Wing M, Compston A (2003) Oligodendroglial-derived stress signals recruit microglia in vitro. *Neuroreport* 14: 1001-1005.

Nicholas RS, Stevens S, Wing MG, Compston DA (2002) Microglia-derived IGF-2 prevents TNFalpha induced death of mature oligodendrocytes in vitro. *J Neuroimmunol* 124: 36-44.

Nicholas RS, Wing MG, Compston A (2001) Nonactivated microglia promote oligodendrocyte precursor survival and maturation through the transcription factor NF-kappa B. *Eur J Neurosci* 13: 959-967.

Niederost BP, Zimmermann DR, Schwab ME, Bandtlow CE (1999) Bovine CNS myelin contains neurite growth-inhibitory activity associated with chondroitin sulfate proteoglycans. *J Neurosci* 19: 8979-8989.

Nimmerjahn A, Kirchhoff F, Helmchen F (2005) Resting microglial cells are highly dynamic surveillants of brain parenchyma in vivo. *Science* 308: 1314-1318.

Noble M (2000) Precursor cell transitions in oligodendrocyte development. *J Cell Biol* 148: 839-842.

Olah M, Amor S, Brouwer N, Vinet J, Eggen B, Biber K, Boddeke HW (2012) Identification of a microglia phenotype supportive of remyelination. *Glia* 60: 306-321.

Palazuelos J, Klingener M, Aguirre A (2014) TGFbeta Signaling Regulates the Timing of CNS Myelination by Modulating Oligodendrocyte Progenitor Cell Cycle Exit through SMAD3/4/FoxO1/Sp1. *J Neurosci* 34: 7917-7930.

Pang Y, Cai Z, Rhodes PG (2003) Disturbance of oligodendrocyte development, hypomyelination and white matter injury in the neonatal rat brain after intracerebral injection of lipopolysaccharide. *Brain Res Dev Brain Res* 140: 205-214.

Pang Y, Fan LW, Tien LT, Dai X, Zheng B, Cai Z, Lin RC, Bhatt A (2013) Differential roles of astrocyte and microglia in supporting oligodendrocyte development and myelination in vitro. *Brain Behav* 3: 503-514.

Pang Y, Zheng B, Fan LW, Rhodes PG, Cai Z (2007) IGF-1 protects oligodendrocyte progenitors against TNFalpha-induced damage by activation of PI3K/Akt and interruption of the mitochondrial apoptotic pathway. *Glia* 55: 1099-1107.

Paolicelli RC, Bolasco G, Pagani F, Maggi L, Scianni M, Panzanelli P, Giustetto M, Ferreira TA, Guiducci E, Dumas L, Ragozzino D, Gross CT (2011) Synaptic pruning by microglia is necessary for normal brain development. *Science* 333: 1456-1458.

Park E, Velumian AA, Fehlings MG (2004) The role of excitotoxicity in secondary mechanisms of spinal cord injury: a review with an emphasis on the implications for white matter degeneration. *J Neurotrauma* 21: 754-774.

Pasquini LA, Millet V, Hoyos HC, Giannoni JP, Croci DO, Marder M, Liu FT, Rabinovich GA, Pasquini JM (2011) Galectin-3 drives oligodendrocyte differentiation to control myelin integrity and function. *Cell Death Differ* 18: 1746-1756.

Peferoen L, Kipp M, van der Valk P, van Noort JM, Amor S (2014) Oligodendrocyte-microglia cross-talk in the central nervous system. *Immunology* 141: 302-313.

Piani D, Fontana A (1994) Involvement of the cystine transport system xc- in the macrophage-induced glutamate-dependent cytotoxicity to neurons. *J Immunol* 152: 3578-3585.

Prineas JW, Kwon EE, Cho ES, Sharer LR, Barnett MH, Oleszak EL, Hoffman B, Morgan BP (2001) Immunopathology of secondary-progressive multiple sclerosis. *Ann Neurol* 50: 646-657.

Rabchevsky AG, Streit WJ (1997) Grafting of cultured microglial cells into the lesioned spinal cord of adult rats enhances neurite outgrowth. *J Neurosci Res* 47: 34-48.

Rathnasamy G, Ling EA, Kaur C (2011) Iron and iron regulatory proteins in amoeboid microglial cells are linked to oligodendrocyte death in hypoxic neonatal rat periventricular white matter through production of proinflammatory cytokines and reactive oxygen/nitrogen species. *J Neurosci* 31: 17982-17995.

Rathore KI, Redensek A, David S (2012) Iron homeostasis in astrocytes and microglia is differentially regulated by TNF-alpha and TGF-beta1. *Glia* 60: 738-750.

Reichert F, Rotshenker S (1999) Galectin-3/MAC-2 in experimental allergic encephalomyelitis. *Exp Neurol* 160: 508-514.

Remington LT, Babcock AA, Zehntner SP, Owens T (2007) Microglial recruitment, activation, and proliferation in response to primary demyelination. *Am J Pathol* 170: 1713-1724.

Rodriguez JP, Coulter M, Miotke J, Meyer RL, Takemaru K, Levine JM (2014) Abrogation of beta-catenin signaling in oligodendrocyte precursor cells reduces glial scarring and promotes axon regeneration after CNS injury. *J Neurosci* 34: 10285-10297.

Rolls A, Shechter R, London A, Segev Y, Jacob-Hirsch J, Amariglio N, Rechavi G, Schwartz M (2008) Two faces of chondroitin sulfate proteoglycan in spinal cord repair: a role in microglia/macrophage activation. *PLoS Med* 5: e171.

Rolls A, Shechter R, Schwartz M (2009) The bright side of the glial scar in CNS repair. *Nat Rev Neurosci* 10: 235-241.

Schafer DP, Lehrman EK, Kautzman AG, Koyama R, Mardinly AR, Yamasaki R, Ransohoff RM, Greenberg ME, Barres BA, Stevens B (2012) Microglia sculpt postnatal neural circuits in an activity and complement-dependent manner. *Neuron* 74: 691-705.

Schonberg DL, McTigue DM (2009) Iron is essential for oligodendrocyte genesis following intraspinal macrophage activation. *Exp Neurol* 218: 64-74.

Schonberg DL, Popovich PG, McTigue DM (2007) Oligodendrocyte generation is differentially influenced by toll-like receptor (TLR) 2 and TLR4-mediated intraspinal macrophage activation. *J Neuropathol Exp Neurol* 66: 1124-1135.

Schulz K, Kroner A, David S (2012) Iron efflux from astrocytes plays a role in remyelination. *J Neurosci* 32: 4841-4847.

Schwartz M, Kipnis J, Rivest S, Prat A (2013) How do immune cells support and shape the brain in health, disease, and aging? *J Neurosci* 33: 17587-17596.

Shigemoto-Mogami Y, Hoshikawa K, Goldman JE, Sekino Y, Sato K (2014) Microglia enhance neurogenesis and oligodendrogenesis in the early postnatal subventricular zone. *J Neurosci* 34: 2231-2243.

Shuman SL, Bresnahan JC, Beattie MS (1997) Apoptosis of microglia and oligodendrocytes after spinal cord contusion in rats. *J Neurosci Res* 50: 798-808.

Siebert JR, Osterhout DJ (2011) The inhibitory effects of chondroitin sulfate proteoglycans on oligodendrocytes. *J Neurochem* 119: 176-188.

Siebert JR, Stelzner DJ, Osterhout DJ (2011) Chondroitinase treatment following spinal contusion injury increases migration of oligodendrocyte progenitor cells. *Exp Neurol* 231: 19-29.

Sierra A, Encinas JM, Deudero JJ, Chancey JH, Enikolopov G, Overstreet-Wadiche LS, Tsirka SE, Maletic-Savatic M (2010) Microglia shape adult hippocampal neurogenesis through apoptosis-coupled phagocytosis. *Cell Stem Cell* 7: 483-495.

Skripuletz T, Miller E, Grote L, Gudi V, Pul R, Voss E, Skuljec J, Moharregh-Khiabani D, Trebst C, Stangel M (2011) Lipopolysaccharide delays demyelination and promotes oligodendrocyte precursor proliferation in the central nervous system. *Brain Behav Immun* 25: 1592-1606.

Smith-Thomas LC, Fok-Seang J, Stevens J, Du JS, Muir E, Faissner A, Geller HM, Rogers JH, Fawcett JW (1994) An inhibitor of neurite outgrowth produced by astrocytes. *J Cell Sci* 107 (Pt 6): 1687-1695.

Smith AM, Dragunow M (2014) The human side of microglia. *Trends Neurosci* 37: 125-135.

Talbott JF, Cao Q, Bertram J, Nkansah M, Benton RL, Lavik E, Whittemore SR (2007) CNTF promotes the survival and differentiation of adult spinal cord-derived oligodendrocyte precursor cells in vitro but fails to promote remyelination in vivo. *Exp Neurol* 204: 485-489.

Talbott JF, Loy DN, Liu Y, Qiu MS, Bunge MB, Rao MS, Whittemore SR (2005) Endogenous Nkx2.2+/Olig2+ oligodendrocyte precursor cells fail to remyelinate the demyelinated adult rat spinal cord in the absence of astrocytes. *Exp Neurol* 192: 11-24

Thorburne SK, Juurlink BH (1996) Low glutathione and high iron govern the susceptibility of oligodendroglial precursors to oxidative stress. *J Neurochem* 67: 1014-1022.

Todorich B, Pasquini JM, Garcia CI, Paez PM, Connor JR (2009) Oligodendrocytes and myelination: the role of iron. *Glia* 57: 467-478.

Totoiu MO, Keirstead HS (2005) Spinal cord injury is accompanied by chronic progressive demyelination. *J Comp Neurol* 486: 373-383.

Tripathi R, McTigue DM (2007) Prominent oligodendrocyte genesis along the border of spinal contusion lesions. *Glia* 55: 698-711.

Ueno M, Fujita Y, Tanaka T, Nakamura Y, Kikuta J, Ishii M, Yamashita T (2013) Layer V cortical neurons require microglial support for survival during postnatal development. *Nat Neurosci* 16: 543-551.

Varnum MM, Ikezu T (2012) The classification of microglial activation phenotypes on neurodegeneration and regeneration in Alzheimer's disease brain. *Arch Immunol Ther Exp (Warsz)* 60: 251-266.

Voss EV, Skuljec J, Gudi V, Skripuletz T, Pul R, Trebst C, Stangel M (2012) Characterisation of microglia during de- and remyelination: can they create a repair promoting environment? *Neurobiol Dis* 45: 519-528.

Wang D, Ichiyama RM, Zhao R, Andrews MR, Fawcett JW (2011) Chondroitinase combined with rehabilitation promotes recovery of forelimb function in rats with chronic spinal cord injury. *J Neurosci* 31: 9332-9344.

Wegiel J, Wisniewski HM, Dziewiatkowski J, Tarnawski M, Kozielski R, Trenkner E, Wiktor-Jedrzejczak W (1998) Reduced number and altered morphology of microglial cells in colony stimulating factor-1-deficient osteopetrotic op/op mice. *Brain Res* 804: 135-139.

Woodruff RH, Fruttiger M, Richardson WD, Franklin RJ (2004) Platelet-derived growth factor regulates oligodendrocyte progenitor numbers in adult CNS and their response following CNS demyelination. *Mol Cell Neurosci* 25: 252-262.

Wu J, Yoo S, Wilcock D, Lytle JM, Leung PY, Colton CA, Wrathall JR (2010) Interaction of NG2(+) glial progenitors and microglia/macrophages from the injured spinal cord. *Glia* 58: 410-422.

Yeo YA, Martinez Gomez JM, Croxford JL, Gasser S, Ling EA, Schwarz H (2012) CD137 ligand activated microglia induces oligodendrocyte apoptosis via reactive oxygen species. *J Neuroinflammation* 9: 173.

Yune TY, Lee JY, Jung GY, Kim SJ, Jiang MH, Kim YC, Oh YJ, Markelonis GJ, Oh TH (2007) Minocycline alleviates death of oligodendrocytes by inhibiting pro-nerve growth factor production in microglia after spinal cord injury. *J Neurosci* 27: 7751-7761.

Zecca L, Youdim MB, Riederer P, Connor JR, Crichton RR (2004) Iron, brain ageing and neurodegenerative disorders. *Nat Rev Neurosci* 5: 863-873.

Zeger M, Popken G, Zhang J, Xuan S, Lu QR, Schwab MH, Nave KA, Rowitch D, D'Ercole AJ, Ye P (2007) Insulin-like growth factor type 1 receptor signaling in the cells of oligodendrocyte lineage is required for normal in vivo oligodendrocyte development and myelination. *Glia* 55: 400-411.

Zhang P, Chebath J, Lonai P, Revel M (2004) Enhancement of oligodendrocyte differentiation from murine embryonic stem cells by an activator of gp130 signaling. *Stem Cells* 22: 344-354.

Zhang SC, Goetz BD, Duncan ID (2003) Suppression of activated microglia promotes survival and function of transplanted oligodendroglial progenitors. *Glia* 41: 191-198..

Zhang Y, Taveggia C, Melendez-Vasquez C, Einheber S, Raine CS, Salzer JL, Brosnan CF, John GR (2006) Interleukin-11 potentiates oligodendrocyte survival and maturation, and myelin formation. *J Neurosci* 26: 12174-12185.

In: Oligodendrocytes
Editor: Dana Swanson
ISBN: 978-1-63483-330-1

Chapter 3

Cell Transplantation for Myelination of Axons in Spinal Cord Repair

Li Yao[*]
Department of Biological Sciences,
Wichita State University, Wichita, KS, US

Abstract

The myelin sheath that is formed by oligodendrocytes (OLs) insulate the axon from electrical activity and allow the rapid conduction of nerve impulses across axons. Direct mechanical injury and pathophysiological changes in secondary injury to the spinal cord cause death of OLs and demyelination of axons. Oligodendrocyte precursors (OPCs) maintain their capability of continuous generation throughout life. The adult central nervous system retains the potential to generate OPCs and the capacity for myelination after spinal cord injury (SCI). OPCs migrate from gray and white matter to the lesion, and after SCI, they differentiate into OLs that eventually myelinate axons. However, the intrinsic capacity for remyelination by OPCs is limited in the adult spinal cord. Focal

[*] Corresponding author: Li Yao, PhD Department of Biological Sciences; Wichita State University; Wichita, KS, USA, 67260; Phone: +001-316-978-6766; Fax: +001-316-978-3772; Email: li.yao@wichita.edu.

delivery of cells, including OPCs, OPCs derived from embryonic stem cells (ECSs) and neural stem cells (NSCs), Schwann cells (SCs), and olfactory-ensheathing cells (OECs), has been investigated to remyelinate axons and promote functional recovery. A biomaterial scaffold that mediates the contact guidance of neural tissue growth and provides a permissive microenvironment for grafted cell growth can act as a vehicle for cell delivery in order to enhance axonal myelination. Improvement of cell transplantation strategies is a promising approach for the effective treatment of SCI clinically.

1. Demyelination of Axons After Spinal Cord Injury

The myelin sheath that is formed by oligodendrocytes (OLs) is a spiral structure around a spinal axon. Each oligodendrocyte forms multiple segments of myelin that wrap around many spinal axons. The myelin sheath insulates the axon from electrical activity, and the segmented structure of the sheath allows for rapid saltatory conduction of nerve impulse across the segments. Spinal cord injury (SCI) is caused by direct mechanical injury and pathophysiological changes in the secondary injury. The initial injury to the spinal cord results in massive tissue destruction, cellular damage, vascular rupture, and hemorrhage. The resulting trauma causes acute death of neurons and glial cells. OLs undergo both necrosis and apoptosis in the lesion. In one study, a rat spinal cord was subjected to a contusion injury. OL cell death was observed within eight hours post-SCI [1]. In another study, after an incomplete midthoracic contusion injury of a rat spinal cord, OL loss followed the same temporal pattern as that of ventral motoneurons (VMNs). The loss of OLs in ventral white matter was significant at the epicenter four hours after SCI [2].

In the secondary injury of a SCI, a cascade of cellular and molecular reactions may progress over several days or weeks [3-5]. A large number of oligodendrocytes undergo apoptosis at sites that are distant to the epicenter of the primary injury. Prominent OL apoptosis was detected in degenerating axon tracts rostral and caudal to the injury site, and the apoptosis lasted for at least three weeks after rats were subjected to a contusion injury [6, 7]. The loss of OLs results in demyelination of spinal axons after SCI. During the first a few weeks after a contusive injury of a cat spinal cord, both partial and full-thickness demyelination can be observed in the lesion of the spinal cord [8]. Wallerian degeneration occurs in the axon stump distal to the site of injury, and demyelination is accompanied by Wallerian degeneration. In one study, a dorsal column cordotomy at the T8 level of rat spinal cord induced Wallerian degeneration in both the corticospinal tract (CST) and the dorsal ascending tract (DAT). Apoptosis of cells including OLs was observed in both tracts throughout cord segments (from T3 to T12) that were analyzed in the study. The delayed cell death began seven days after injury and peaked at 14 days for the DAT and 28 days for the CST [7]. In another study, following contusion injury of a rat spinal cord, cell apoptosis was detected in the white matter for long distances remotely located from the center of the lesion, and OL death was maximal at eight days post-SCI. Activated microglia were found in the same regions as the apoptotic OLs. This study suggests that the loss of trophic support after axonal degeneration and microglial activation resulted in apoptosis [9].

Many factors cause the loss of OLs in the lesion environment. Glutamate is an essential excitatory neurotransmitter regulating functions of neural tissue. Following rat SCI, the release of glutamate was toxic to OLs. An *in vivo* study investigated the toxicity of glutamate to OLs in the rat spinal cord. Glutamate was administered into rat spinal cords and caused a reduction in OL density. Most glutamate-induced OL death occurs within 24 hours after exposure [10]. A small amount of free radicals, such as superoxide and hydroxyl, is produced by the mitochondrial electron transport chain and the microsomal cytochrome P-450 system. Nitric oxide (NO) is generated by the vascular endothelium and neurons in the central nervous system (CNS). Immediately following contusion injury of the spinal cord, the NO level increased significantly and then gradually decreased between one and 12 days after injury [11]. Ischemia and reperfusion also enhanced the generation of free radicals in the wounded spinal cord. Nitrosative and oxidative stress also can trigger mitochondrial fragmentation and induce cell death [12, 13].

Cysteine proteases are involved in multiple cellular processes such as apoptosis, inflammation, and abnormal immune responses. Cysteine proteases play critical roles in cell death in acute and chronic SCI. Caspases are the main cysteine proteases for execution of apoptosis and are involved in OL apoptosis in SCI. In one study, the activation of caspases were investigated from one hour to seven days after contusion injury induced by a weight-drop method in the rat. Caspases 3, 8, and 9 were primarily activated in neurons and OLs, and intrathecal injection of the caspase inhibitor improved rat locomotor function [14]. Calpains are the Ca2+-dependent cysteine proteases and can cause both necrotic and apoptotic death in SCI [15, 16]. In an *in vivo* study, the calpain content and activity were examined post-SCI. Administration of the calpain-specific inhibitor to injured rat spinal cords continuously for 24 hours inhibited calpain activity and other factors that lead to apoptosis in the lesion and surrounding areas. Results obtained from this animal model of SCI suggest that the calpain inhibitor can provide neuroprotection in patients with SCI [15].

2. Response of Endogenous Oligodendrocyte Precursors to Demyelination after Spinal Cord Injury

In the developing CNS, oligodendrocyte precursors (OPCs) are generated in the subventricular zone (SVZ) and migrate long distances to participate in the formation of white matter [17, 18]. OL progenitors maintain the capability of continuous generation throughout life. The adult CNS retains the potential to generate OPCs and the capacity for myelination after SCI [19]. Endogenous OPCs, which are present throughout adult gray and white matter, mediate remyelination post-SCI. In response to demyelination, OPCs proliferate and migrate into the demyelinated zone [20]. Adult OPCs typically express nerve/glial antigen 2 (NG2) or platelet-derived growth factor receptor (PDGFRα). New progenitor cells can also be produced in the SVZ, and migrate and participate in myelination after injury [21, 22]. Though remyelination may improve axonal conduction, the adult CNS has a limited capacity to spontaneously remyelinate [21-27]. Though SCI induces proliferation of local progenitors, most cells are astrocytes, and few cells are OLs [28, 29]. In one study, rats received bromodeoxyuridine (BrdU) injections during the first week after contusion injury of the spinal cord [29]. Then the animals were perfused within two hours for acute studies and at six weeks for chronic studies. Immunohistochemical assay showed that cell proliferation in the residual white matter was increased one to seven days after SCI, peaking on day 3. Dividing cells include oligodendrocytes, astrocytes, microglia/macrophages, and NG2(+) precursors. By six weeks, some cells that had been labeled two to four days after SCI were still present, but very few of these cells expressed NG2.

Differentiation of OPCs is regulated by growth factors (PDGF, NT-3, BDNF, CNTF, bFGF), notch signaling, substrate signaling, and chemokines [17, 19, 30, 31]. Growth factors such as PDGF and bFGF can promote the division of OPCs and increase cell number, while TGF-β inhibits the proliferation of OPCs and induces cell maturation. It was reported that the differentiation of OPCs *in vitro* is inhibited by notch signaling [32], and therefore, notch signaling may regulate the differentiation of OLs spatially and temporally in the central nervous system [33]. The proliferative response of spinal cord OPCs to PDGF depends on the chemokine CXCL1 [34, 35]. CXCL1 inhibited the migration of OPCs and widespread dispersal of post-natal precursors observed in slices of CXCR2 knockout animals [30].

Changes in the microenvironment during recovery from SCI may regulate the fate of NG2-expressing progenitors. The NG2-expressing progenitors showed a shift between astroglial scar formation and the generation of myelinating OLs post-SCI [36]. One study showed that NG2 progenitors born 24 hours after SCI mainly generated scar-forming astrocytes, while NG2 progenitors born seven days after injury generated mature, myelinating OLs [36].

The remyelination processes of spinal cord axons post-SCI show patterns of both central- and peripheral-like myelin. In addition to OPCs, peripheral Schwann cells (SCs) regenerate and migrate to the injury site post-SCI and are involved in the myelin formation of spinal cord axons [37, 38]. In one study, the distribution of peripheral and central myelin proteins at the lesion of 13 postmortem chronically injured human spinal cords were studied by immunohistochemical methods. This study found that SCs contributed to the restoration of myelin sheaths around some spinal axons [38]. Some SCs that form the peripheral-like myelin are derived from progenitor cells in the CNS [39-41]. When neural precursor cells derived from adult human brain tissue removed during surgery were cultured, a small number of cells showed the properties of SCs. When the neural precursor cells were transplanted into the demyelinated adult rat spinal cord, extensive remyelination was formed and showed a peripheral myelin pattern similar to Schwann cell-formed myelination.

3. Cell Implantation for Axon Remyelination After Spinal Cord Injury

OLs undergo both necrosis and apoptosis shortly after SCI and the cell death results in demyelination and the loss of appropriate axonal conduction. In response to demyelination, oligodendrocyte precursor cells are recruited from gray and white matter and migrate to the lesion to myelinate the regenerated axon; however, the intrinsic capacity for oligodendroglial replacement and remyelination is limited in the adult spinal cord. The differentiation of OPCs into the myelinating OLs is insufficient [20, 42]. A number of cell types, including OPCs, OPCs derived from embryonic stem cells and neural stem cells (NSCs), SCs and olfactory-ensheathing cells (OECs), have been investigated for focal delivery to remyelinate axons.

3.1. Oligodendrocyte Precursors

OPCs have demonstrated the capacity to myelinate axons after they were transplanted into a demyelinated CNS. In one study, they were isolated from the fetal human forebrain and adult white matter. These cells were grafted into the forebrains of newborn shiverer mice, which are deficient in myelin basic protein (MBP). Both fetal and adult OPCs mediated the extensive and robust myelination of congenitally dysmyelinated mice brain [43]. The transplantation of OPCs can also enhance remyelination and functional recovery after SCI [44, 45]. In one study, OPCs were isolated from newborn rat pups and transplanted into the rat spinal cord with contusion injury [44]. Immunohistochemical analysis showed the survival, proliferation, and migration of implanted cells. The animals transplanted with OPCs showed significant improvement in locomotor function and motor-evoked potential (MEP). In another study, OPCs that were isolated from the spinal cord of adult Fischer 344 rats and infected with retroviruses expressing CNTF were transplanted into the contused thoracic spinal cord of adult rats nine days after injury [45]. Results showed that the grafted OPCs survived and were integrated into the injured spinal cord seven weeks after transplantation. The central myelin sheaths were formed around the axons by the grafted OPCs in the injured spinal cord. Transplantation of OPCs expressing CNTF significantly enhanced the recovery of hind limb locomotor function.

A number of studies have isolated OPCs from human tissue [46-49]. A previous work demonstrated the possibility of transplantation of OPCs to myelinate axons post-SCI clinically. One study showed that tissue fragments obtained from the brains and spinal cords of ten-week-old human fetuses provided the source of OPCs. These tissues were transplanted into the brains of newborn shiverer mutant mice. OPCs migrated out from these fragments and myelinated axons *in vivo* [50].

3.2. Embryonic Stem-Derived Oligodendrocyte Precursors

Though OPCs demonstrated the potential to myelinate axons post-SCI, the application of human OPCs in spinal cord repair has been restricted by their limited availability in embryonic human tissue. It is also difficult to provide a sufficient number of cells for transplantation because of the limited proliferation potential of cultured OPCs. OPCs derived from human embryonic stem cells (hESCs) provided an alternative source of cells to treat SCI [51-53]. The high-purity OPCs derived from hESCs were transplanted rats seven days or ten months after spinal cord injury [53]. The transplanted hESCs-derived OPCs survived, were redistributed over short distances, and differentiated into oligodendrocytes. The transplanted cells enhanced remyelination and substantially improved locomotor ability for the rat seven days after SCI. However, animals that received transplantation of cells did not show functional recovery a few months post-injury. The myelination function of hESC-derived OPCs has also been investigated in an animal model with a completely transected spinal cord. The grafted hESC-derived OPCs survived and migrated in the damaged neural tissue, and differentiated into mature OLs. Animals treated with the cells showed improved locomotor function based on the evaluation of Basso-Beattie-Bresnahan scores [52].

3.3. Schwann Cells

SCs form the myelin sheaths for peripheral nerves and are also involved in the re-myelination of axons in SCI. SCs regenerated and migrated to the injury site, and participated in the regeneration process post-SCI [38]. Because they can be easily isolated from the peripheral nerve and cultured *in vitro*, SCs are a valuable source of cells for autografts to facilitate remyelination in spinal cord repair. The remyelinating capacity of SCs for the axons of a spinal cord has been demonstrated in a number of studies of SCI [38, 54-56]. In one study, rat SCs were transplanted into the spinal cords of myelin mutant mice. From 2 to 18 weeks after implantation, remyelination of spinal axons by SCs was observed in the dorsal columns. This study suggested that cultured SCs can retain their potential to myelinate axons when they are transplanted into the spinal cord of a xenogenic host [57]. In one study, SCs were transplanted into the contused adult rat spinal cord at one week post-injury. The myelination of numerous axons by the grafted SCs was observed in the wounded spinal cord. However, grafted SCs did not migrate after injection. Most grafted SCs remained at the immediate site of injection over time. The poor migration ability of SCs from their original site of injection limited their potential to remyelinate axons after SCI [Guest et al., 2005; Totoiu and Kierstead, 2005].

3.4. Olfactory-Ensheating Cells

The olfactory nerve continuously regenerates in the CNS of adult mammals. OECs ensheath the olfactory nerve and have the potency to support the regeneration of olfactory axons in mammals [54]. They are relatively easy to obtain compared with hESCs and human OPCs, because they can be isolated from the biopsy of the olfactory mucosa. OECs have been investigated for their ability to myelinate axons of SCI in a number of studies [58-64]. These studies demonstrated the effect of grafted OECs for axon remyelination, neuroprotection, facilitation of axonal regrowth, and functional improvement in the treatment of incomplete and complete SCI.

In one study, after cultured OEC cells that were isolated from an adult rat olfactory bulb, the cells were injected into the transected rat upper cervical corticospinal tract [60]. The grafted cells induced unbranched, elongative growth of the cut corticospinal axons. Axons grew through the transplant and continued to regenerate into the denervated caudal host tract. Further study showed that introduction of therapeutic genes into the OEC cells can promote the function of cells in neural regeneration. In one study, cultured OEC cells were transduced by adenoviral vectors encoding neurotrophin-3. Then the cells were transplanted into an adult Fischer 344 rat spinal cord immediately after unilateral cervical (C4) corticospinal tract (CST) transection. Results showed that genetic modification can enhance the effect of OECs on promoting long-distance maintenance and regeneration of lesioned adult CST axons [65]. It was reported that human OECs can also remyelinate demyelinated spinal cord axons [66, 67]. Human OECs were isolated from olfactory bulbs during surgery for tumor removal. The cells were transplanted into a focal area containing demyelinated axons in the rat spinal cord.

This study showed that OECs were able to remyelinate demyelinated axons after they were transplanted into experimentally induced demyelinating lesions in a rat spinal cord.

4. Biomaterial-Based Cell Transplantation for Axon Remyelination

Though cell transplantation is potentially an effective approach to remyelinate regenerating axons and restore spinal cord function [68, 69], the microenvironment that transplanted cells will encounter is unfavorable for their survival. The development of implantable biomaterial has offered a promising solution for the treatment of wounded neural tissue because potentially it can generate a permissive environment for the growth of grafted cells. *In vivo* studies have shown that transected or partially wounded spinal cord reconstructed by bridging the gap with neural conduits or filling the defect with hydrogels exhibited improved neural regeneration [70-72]. A biomaterial scaffold that mediates the contact guidance of neural tissue growth can also act as a vehicle for cell delivery to enhance axonal myelination [73-76]. Biomaterial scaffolds may also serve as a carrier for the delivery of cells to treat the injured spinal cord and to improve the survival of transplanted cells [77, 78]. By targeting cell transplantation to the lesion and therapy, cells encapsulated in the biomaterials should generate proper function after transplantation. Biomaterial scaffolds for this application must have appropriate mechanical durability, pore size, capsule consistency, degradation features, and low immunogenicity [79].

Nanofibers have a high surface-to-volume ratio, and this high surface area can enhance the capacity for cell adhesion [80, 81]. Nanofibers can be generated by electrospinning, and the graft of nanofiber scaffolds may enhance neural regeneration because nanofibers mimic the extracellular matrix and provide guidance for axonal growth at nano-levels. Previous studies have shown that electrospun aligned fibers can guide the growth of dorsal root ganglia (DRG) neurons *in vitro* [82-84]. Nanofibers can also enhance axonal regeneration when they were grafted into the injured spinal cord and peripheral nerve [85-88]. The neurotrophic and neuroprotective effects of neuroglia are critical in neural regeneration. Nanofibers can also potentially deliver NSCs to the lesion of SCI to promote myelination and regeneration of axons. An *in vitro* study reported the interaction of multiple glial cell populations including astrocytes, OPCs, and OLs with aligned nanofibers [89]. The parallel nanofibers induced an oriented growth of astrocytes, and the growth, elongation and maturation of OPCs required prealigned astrocytes. This study suggested that the scaffolds of nanofibers are implantable and could be an effective approach to reconstruct glial circuitry in SCI.

Micro- and nano-scale carriers synthesized from various natural and synthetic polymers have been investigated to encapsulate biomolecules or therapeutic cells. Biomolecules encapsulated in particles may generate a significant biological effect through a small volume [90-92]. Different from the hydrogel approach, which is particularly suitable to filling a neural defect, microspheres can be delivered to a lesion without significant neural defect because the size of the microspheres are relatively small. Cell delivery by microspheres and transplantation to the targeted tissue may be an efficient approach for cell therapy. Previous studies showed that microspheres were suitable for stem cell growth and can potentially deliver stem cells to the injured area for tissue regeneration [93, 94]. Microspheres may provide an optimal condition for the delivered cells to adapt to the hostile environment in the lesion of SCI. Because of the biodegradable and biocompatible properties, natural polymers are strongly favored for the cell delivery. In one study, collagen microspheres were fabricated using the water-in-oil emulsion technique and crosslinked with 1-ethyl-3-(3-dimethylaminopropryl) carbodiimide (EDC) [95]. The oligodendrocyte progenitor cells isolated from neonatal rats grew and differentiated on the microspheres. OPCs on the microspheres were co-cultured with DRGs. Results showed that the OLs grown on microspheres extended the processes that wrapped the axons of DRG neurons, and the formation of myelin sheath was observed in the co-culture. This study demonstrated the feasibility of using collagen microspheres to deliver OPCs to myelinate axons in SCI and that the collagen-based microspheres will cause little damage to the healthy tissue after implantation because of its elastic property.

In vivo studies have shown that implantation of biomaterial scaffolds seeded with stem cells such as NSCs, MSCs, and hESCs can improve axonal regeneration, reduce glial scar formation, and promote functional recovery post-SCI. Glial-restricted precursor cells (GRPs) that were isolated from an embryonic day-14 rat spinal cord were able to differentiate into both oligodendrocytes and astrocytes [96]. GRPs formed normal-appearing central myelin around axons of cultured DRG neurons. Infected with retroviruses expressing BDNF and NT3, GRPs were transplanted into contused adult thoracic spinal cord nine days after injury. Six weeks after transplantation, the grafted GRPs differentiated into mature oligodendrocytes and formed myelin sheaths around the axons. Recovery of hind limb locomotor function was also significantly enhanced for rats grafted with GRPs expressing BDNF and NT3. To enhance remyelination and axon regeneration, biomaterials with Schwann cells were grafted into the injured spinal cord, and results were encouraging

[97-100]. After the transplantation of autologous sciatic nerve segments were transplanted into the thoracic region of a rat spinal cord, axons grew into the grafts. Retrograde tracing assay showed that some axons in the grafts originated from intrinsic CNS neurons with their cell bodies in nearby segments of the spinal cord and that others arose from DRG at the level of the grafts. However, no obvious functional improvement was observed [101]. In recent studies, synthetic neural conduits containing SCs were investigated to bridge the injured spinal cord. In one study, SC-seeded channels were implanted into hemisected adult rat thoracic spinal cords. One month after treatment, significant numbers of regenerating axons grew into the channels and crossed the distal interface into the caudal host cord. Enhanced myelination of axons in the regenerated tissue cable was also observed [97].

The co-culture of DRG neurons and oligodendrocyte precursor cells is the general model for myelination studies. The intimate interaction between axons and oligodendrocytes that direct myelination formation of the regenerated axons is a complicated process [102-104]. Additionally, the nerve growth factor (NGF) in the cell culture medium is required for the survival of embryonic DRG neurons can negatively affect the myelination function of oligodendrocytes to the axons [102, 103]. The fetal bovine serum in the cell culture medium can significantly increase the non-specific cells, which can make the analysis of myelination more complicated [103]. A recent study revealed a neuron-free model to investigate myelination using nanofibers. It was shown that oligodendrocytes can myelinate electrospun fibers of synthetic polymers [105]. OPCs interact with nanofibers in a relatively isolated environment using the optimal cell culture medium targeting the myelination process. Such a neuron-free model allows the myelination study to focus on the interaction of particular biological molecules and OPCs.

The function of a particular biological molecule in the myelination process can be studied by incorporating it into fibers. In one study, nanofibers were fabricated by a polycaprolactone (PCL) and gelatin copolymer [106]. PCL was investigated as a biomaterial scaffold for neural regeneration because of its biodegradable and biocompatible properties [87, 88]. Gelatin, a heterogeneous mixture of polypeptides formed by thermal denaturation of collagen, maintains the biological property of collagen. Gelatin in the nanofibers decreased the contact angle of the electrospun fibers. Results showed that both PCL nanofibers and PCL-gelatin copolymer nanofibers can support OPC growth and differentiation [106]. The differentiated OLs extend multiple processes along the nanofibers and wrapped the nanofibers. OLs formed significantly more myelinated segments on the PCL-gelatin copolymer nanofibers than those on PCL nanofibers alone. This study suggested that the implantation of electrospun PCL-gelatin copolymer nanofibers with OPCs may enhance the myelination of regenerated axons. It also showed the effect of biological molecules in the nanofibers on myelination function of OPCs.

5. Clinical Application of Cell Transplantation for Myelination in Spinal Cord Repair

A number of clinical trials for the repair of injured spinal cords by cell-based therapy have been conducted. To improve myelination and restore the functional recovery of the injured spinal cord, OECs have been transplanted into the patient in clinical trials. Other cell types including Schwann cells, hESC-derived OPCs, and NSC-derived OPCs have also been proposed for clinical trials. To ensure that clinical trials for SCI repair are performed properly, standards for the appropriate conduct of clinical trials were suggested by the International Campaign for Cures for SCI Paralysis (ICCP) guidelines [107-110].

5.1. Application of Olfactory-Ensheating Cell Transplantation

Transplantation of OEC cell into SCI has been conducted in a few clinical studies; however, the therapeutic effect of this treatment was discrepant in different clinical trials [111-114]. MacKay-Sim, et al. [111] isolated OECs from the nasal mucosa of six patients with chronic SCI. The cells were cultured and transplanted back into the injured spinal cords. The trial was a Phase I/IIa design, and the aim of the study was to test the feasibility and safety of transplantation of autologous OECs into the injured spinal cord in human paraplegia. All patients that received the cell transplantation did not show adverse effects after surgery. There were no significant functional changes in any patients and no neuropathic pain three years after transplantation. However, one patient with transplanted cells showed an improvement over three segments in light-touch and pin-prick sensitivity bilaterally, anteriorly, and posteriorly.

Different from the findings of MacKay-Sim, et al., the functional improvement in patients with cell implantation was reported by another research group. In that study, olfactory mucosa autografts (OMAs) were transplanted into seven patients with traumatically injured spinal cords. The authors conveyed that two patients reported return of sensation in their bladders, one of these patients regained voluntary contraction of the anal sphincter, two of the seven ASIA A patients became ASIA C, and every patient had improvement in ASIA motor scores [112]. In a following study, OMAs were transplanted into 20 patients with chronic, sensorimotor complete, or motor complete SCI [115]. OMAs were transplanted into 1.3- to 4-cm lesions at C4-T12 neurological levels after a partial scar was removed. The ASIA Impairment Scale (AIS) improved in 11 of 20 patients, and the improvements included new voluntary electromyography (EMG) responses (15 patients) and somatosensory-evoked potentials (SSEPs) (4 patients). This study indicated that OMA transplantation is a feasible and relatively safe procedure and that it may be beneficial in people with chronic SCI when combined with post-operative rehabilitation.

One study involved a large group of patients and the fetal OEC transplantation for chronic SCI. The authors here reported partially improved neurological functions including motor, light touch, and pin prick [114]. However, Dobkin et al., found unreported complications in SCI patients who received OEC transplantation in those studies. Among seven patients, five had complications including meningitis [116].

5.2. Application of Schwann Cell Transplantation

Transplantation of SCs that are isolated from the autologous peripheral nerve for the human central nervous system repair was proposed previously [117]. A clinical trial involving the transplantation of autologous SCs into the injured spinal cords of four patients with chronic SCI was conducted. In this study, purified SCs used for transplantation were isolated from sural nerves of the patients and cultured without the use of any specific mitogenic or growth factors. One year after transplantation, none of the patients was found to have any adverse effects such as infection, neurological deterioration, or other related clinical problems. However, only one patient with incomplete SCI showed motor and sensory improvement [118]. This study suggested that autologous SC transplantation is safe for the treatment of selected SCI patients, though it does not show beneficial effects.

In the Miami Project, several clinical trials and clinical studies are being evaluated for patients with acute or chronic spinal cord injuries. These trials are attempting to test the safety and efficacy of different neuroprotective, repairative, or modulatory interventions. The Miami Project has submitted an application to the Food and Drug Administration (FDA) for permission to begin a Phase I clinical trial that will evaluate the safety of autologous human SC transplantation into patients with spinal cord injury. This trial will focus on safety outcomes and risk minimization, because SCs will be directly delivered into the spinal cord using a needle in the treatment procedure. A biopsy of a nerve in one leg of the patient will be performed in order to obtain SCs, which will be cultured for three to five weeks for proliferation and purification. Then a surgery will be conducted to transplant the cells into the site of spinal cord injury. The patients will be followed for one year after the transplantation surgery, and the patient's neurologic status, medical status, pain symptoms, and muscle spasticity will be evaluated (http://www.miamiproject.miami.edu).

References

[1] Liu, XZ; Xu, XM; Hu, R; Du, C; Zhang, SX; McDonald, JW; Don,g HX; Wu, YJ; Fan, GS; Jacquin, MF; Hsu, CY; Choi, DW. Neuronal and glial apoptosis after traumatic spinal cord injury. *J Neurosci,* 1997;17:5395–5406.

[2] Grossman, SD; Rosenberg, LJ; Wrathall, JR. Temporal-spatial pattern of acute neuronal and glial loss after spinal cord contusion. *Exp Neurol,* 2001;168:273–282.

[3] Privat, A. Pathophysiology and treatment of spinal cord injury. *Bull. Acad. Natl Med.,* 2005; 189:1109–1117.

[4] Schwab, JM; Brechtel, K; Mueller, CA; Failli, V; Kaps, HP; Tuli, SK; Schluesener, HJ. Experimental strategies to promote spinal cord regeneration–an integrative perspective. *Prog. Neurobiol.* 2006; 78:91–116.

[5] Park, E; Velumian, AA; Fehlings, MG. The role of excitotoxicity in secondary mechanisms of spinal cord injury: a review with an emphasis on the implications for white matter degeneration. *J. Neurotrauma.,* 2004; 21:754–774.

[6] Crowe, MJ; Bresnahan, JC; Shuman, SL; Masters, JN; Beattie, MS. Apoptosis and delayed degeneration after spinal cord injury in rats and monkeys. *Nat Med,* 1997;3:73–76.

[7] Warden, P; Bamber, NI; Li, H; Esposito, A; Ahmad, KA; Hsu, CY; Xu, XM. Delayed glial cell death following wallerian degeneration in white matter tracts after spinal cord dorsal column cordotomy in adult rats. *Exp Neurol,* 2001;168:213–224.

[8] Griffiths, IR; McCulloch, MC. Nerve fibres in spinal cord impact injuries. Part 1. Changes in the myelin sheath during the initial 5 weeks. *J Neurol Sci.,* 1983;58:335-49.

[9] Shuman, SL; Bresnahan, JC; Beattie, MS. Apoptosis of microglia and oligodendrocytes after spinal cord contusion in rats. *J Neurosci Res.* 1997;50:798-808.

[10] Xu, GY; Hughes, MG; Ye, Z; Hulsebosch, CE; McAdoo, DJ. Concentrations of glutamate released following spinal cord injury kill oligodendrocytes in the spinal cord. *Exp Neurol.*, 2004;187:329-36.

[11] Nakahara, S; Yone, K; Setoguchi, T; Yamaura, I; Arishima, Y; Yoshino, S; Komiya S. Changes in nitric oxide and expression of nitric oxide synthase in spinal cord after traumatic injury in rats. *J Neurotrauma,* 2002; 11: 1467–1474.

[12] Barsoum, MJ; Yuan, H; Gerencser, AA; Liot, G; Kushnareva, Y; Gräber, S; Kovacs, I; Lee, WD; Waggoner, J; Cui, J; White, AD; Bossy, B; Martinou, JC; Youle, RJ; Lipton, SA; Ellisman, MH; Perkins, GA; Bossy-Wetzel, E. Nitric oxide-induced mitochondrial fission is regulated by dynamin-related GTPases in neurons. *EMBO J.* 2006; 25:3900–3911.

[13] Liot, G, Bossy, B; Lubitz, S; Kushnareva, Y; Sejbuk, N; Bossy-Wetzel, E. Complex II inhibition by 3-NP causes mitochondrial fragmentation and neuronal cell death via an NMDA- and ROS-dependent pathway. *Cell Death Differ.* 2009; 16:899–909.

[14] Knoblach, SM; Huang, X; VanGelderen, J; Calva-Cerqueira, D; Faden, AI. Selective caspase activation may contribute to neurological dysfunction after experimental spinal cord trauma. *J Neurosci Res.* 2005;80:369-80.

[15] Ray, SK; Matzelle, DD; Wilford, GG; Hogan, EL; Banik, NL. Inhibition of calpain mediated apoptosis by E-64-d reduced immediate early gene (IEG) expression and reactive astrogliosis in the lesion and penumbra following spinal cord injury in rats. *Brain Res* 2001;916:115–126.

[16] Ray, SK; Hogan, EL; Banik, NL. Calpain in the pathophysiology of spinal cord injury: neuroprotection with calpain inhibitors. *Brain Res* Rev 2003;42:169–185

[17] Baumann, N; Pham-Dinh, D. Biology of oligodendrocyte and myelin in the mammalian central nervous system. *Physiol Rev.* 2001;81:871-927.

[18] García-Verdugo, JM; Doetsch, F; Wichterle, H; Lim DA; Alvarez-Buylla, A. Architecture and cell types of the adult subventricular zone: in search of the stem cells. *J Neurobiol.* 1998;36:234-48.
[19] Horner, PJ; Gage, FH. Regenerating the damaged central nervous system. *Nature*. 2000;407:963-70.
[20] Almad, A; Sahinkaya, FR; McTigue, DM. Oligodendrocyte fate after spinal cord injury. *Neurotherapeutics* 2011, 8:262–273.
[21] Franklin, RJ; Blakemore, WF. Glial-cell transplantation and plasticity in the O-2A lineage--implications for CNS repair. *Trends Neurosci.* 1995;18:151-6.
[22] Franklin, RJ; Blakemore, WF. To what extent is oligodendrocyte progenitor migration a limiting factor in the remyelination of multiple sclerosis lesions? *Mult Scler.* 1997;3:84-7.
[23] Blakemore, WF; Franklin, RJ. Transplantation options for therapeutic central nervous system remyelination. *Cell Transplant*. 2000;9:289-94.
[24] Blight, AR; Young, W. Central axons in injured cat spinal cord recover electrophysiological function following remyelination by Schwann cells. *J Neurol Sci*. 1989;91:15-34.
[25] Gilson, J; Blakemore, WF. Failure of remyelination in areas of demyelination produced in the spinal cord of old rats. *Neuropathol Appl Neurobiol.* 1993;19:173-81.
[26] Blakemore, WF; Keirstead, HS. The origin of remyelinating cells in the central nervous system. *J Neuroimmunol.* 1999;98:69-76.
[27] Ludwin, SK; Bakker, DA. Can oligodendrocytes attached to myelin proliferate? *J Neurosci.* 1988 Apr;8(4):1239-44.
[28] Shibuya, S; Miyamoto, O; Itano, T; Mori, S; Norimatsu, H. Temporal progressive antigen expression in radial glia after contusive spinal cord injury in adult rats. *Glia*. 2003, 15;42:172-83.
[29] Zai, LJ; Wrathall JR. Cell proliferation and replacement following contusive spinal cord injury. *Glia* 2005, 50 : 247 – 257.
[30] Tsai, HH; Frost, E; To, V; Robinson, S; Ffrench-Constant, C; Geertman, R; Ransohoff, RM; Miller, RH. The chemokine receptor CXCR2 controls positioning of oligodendrocyte precursors in developing spinal cord by arresting their migration. *Cell.* 2002;110:373-83.
[31] David, S; Lacroix, S. Molecular approaches to spinal cord repair. *Annu Rev Neurosci.* 2003;26:411-40.
[32] Wang, S; Sdrulla, AD; diSibio, G; Bush G; Nofziger D; Hicks C; Weinmaster G; Barres BA. Notch receptor activation inhibits oligodendrocyte differentiation. *Neuron* 1998, 21, 63–75.

[33] Popko B. Notch signaling: a rheostat regulating oligodendrocyte differentiation? *Dev Cell.* 2003;5:668-9.

[34] Robinson, S; Tani, M; Strieter, RM; Ransohoff, RM; Miller, RH. The chemokine growth related oncogene-alpha promotes spinal cord precursor proliferation. *J. Neurosci.,* 1998;18:10457-63.

[35] Wu, Q; Miller, RH; Ransohoff, RM; Robinson, S; Bu J; Nishiyama, A. Elevated levels of the chemokine GRO-1 correlate with elevated oligodendrocyte progenitor proliferation in the jimpy mutant. *J Neurosci.* 2000;20:2609-17.

[36] Sellers, DL; Maris, DO; Horner, PJ. Postinjury niches induce temporal shifts in progenitor fates to direct lesion repair after spinal cord injury. *J Neurosci.* 2009;29:6722-33.

[37] Gilson, J; Blakemore, WF. Neuropathol Appl Neurobiol. Failure of remyelination in areas of demyelination produced in the spinal cord of old rats. 1993;19:173-81.

[38] Guest, JD; Hiester, ED; Bunge, RP. Demyelination and Schwann cell responses adjacent to injury epicenter cavities following chronic human spinal cord injury. *Exp Neurol.* 2005;192:384-93.

[39] Akiyama, Y; Honmou, O; Kato, T, Uede, T, Hashi, K, Kocsis, JD. Transplantation of clonal neural precursor cells derived from adult human brain establishes functional peripheral myelin in the rat spinal cord. *Experimental neurology,* 2001;167:27–39.

[40] Keirstead, HS; Ben-Hur, T; Rogister, B; O'Leary, MT; Dubois-Dalcq, M; Blakemore, WF. Polysialylated neural cell adhesion molecule-positive CNS precursors generate both oligodendrocytes and Schwann cells to remyelinate the CNS after transplantation. *J Neurosci,* 1999;19:7529–7536.

[41] Mujtaba, T; Mayer-Proschel, M; Rao, MS. A common neural progenitor for the CNS and PNS. *Developmental biology,* 1998;200:1–15.

[42] Levine, JM; Reynolds, R. Activation and proliferation of endogenous oligodendrocyte precursor cells during ethidium bromide-induced demyelination. *Exp Neurol.* 1999;160:333-47.

[43] Windrem, MS; Nunes, MC; Rashbaum, WK; Schwartz, TH; Goodman, RA; McKhann, G 2nd; Roy, NS; Goldman, SA. Fetal and adult human oligodendrocyte progenitor cell isolates myelinate the congenitally dysmyelinated brain. *Nat Med.* 2004;10:93-7.

[44] Bambakidis, NC; Miller, RH. Transplantation of oligodendrocyte precursors and sonic hedgehog results in improved function and white

matter sparing in the spinal cords of adult rats after contusion. *Spine J.* 2004;4:16-26.

[45] Cao, Q; He, Q; Wang, Y; Cheng, X; Howard, RM; Zhang, Y; DeVries, WH; Shields, CB, Magnuson, DS; Xu, XM; Kim, DH; Whittemore, SR. Transplantation of ciliary neurotrophic factor-expressing adult oligodendrocyte precursor cells promotes remyelination and functional recovery after spinal cord injury. *J Neurosci.* 2010;30:2989-3001.

[46] Miron, VE; Jung, CG; Kim, HJ; Kennedy, TE; Soliven, B; Antel, JP. FTY720 modulates human oligodendrocyte progenitor process extension and survival. *Ann Neurol.* 2008;63:61-71.

[47] Roy, NS; Wang, S; Harrison-Restelli, C; Benraiss, A; Fraser, RA; Gravel, M; Braun, PE; Goldman, SA. Identification, isolation, and promoter-defined separation of mitotic oligodendrocyte progenitor cells from the adult human subcortical white matter. *J Neurosci.* 1999;19:9986-95.

[48] Ruffini, F; Arbour, N; Blain, M; Olivier, A; Antel, JP. Distinctive properties of human adult brain-derived myelin progenitor cells. *Am J Pathol.* 2004;165:2167-75.

[49] Windrem MS, Roy NS, Wang J, Nunes M, Benraiss A, Goodman R, McKhann GM 2nd, Goldman SA. Progenitor cells derived from the adult human subcortical white matter disperse and differentiate as oligodendrocytes within demyelinated lesions of the rat brain. *J Neurosci Res.* 2002;69:966-75.

[50] Seilhean D, Gansmüller A, Baron-Van Evercooren A, Gumpel M, Lachapelle F. Myelination by transplanted human and mouse central nervous system tissue after long-term cryopreservation. *Acta Neuropathol.* 1996;91:82-8.

[51] Erceg, S; Ronaghi, M; Oria, M; Roselló, MG; Aragó, MA; Lopez, MG; Radojevic, I; Moreno-Manzano, V; Rodríguez-Jiménez, FJ; Bhattacharya, SS; Cordoba, J; Stojkovic, M. Transplanted oligodendrocytes and motoneuron progenitors generated from human embryonic stem cells promote locomotor recovery after spinal cord transection. *Stem Cells* 2010; 28:1541–1549.

[52] Nistor, GI; Totoiu, MO; Haque, N; Carpenter, MK; Keirstead, HS. Human embryonic stem cells differentiate into oligodendrocytes in high purity and myelinate after spinal cord transplantation. *Glia* 2005; 49:385–396.

[53] Keirstead, HS; Nistor, G; Bernal, G; Totoiu, M; Cloutier, F; Sharp, K; Steward, O. Human embryonic stem cell-derived oligodendrocyte

progenitor cell transplants remyelinate and restore locomotion after spinal cord injury. *J Neurosci* 2005;25:4694–705.

[54] Pinzon, A; Calancie, B; Oudega, M; Noga, BR. Conduction of impulses by axons regenerated in a Schwann cell graft in the transected adult rat thoracic spinal cord. *J Neurosci Res.* 2001; 64: 533–41.

[55] Pearse, DD; Sanchez, AR; Pereira, FC; Andrade, CM; Puzis, R; Pressman, Y; Golden, K; Kitay, BM; Blits, B; Wood, PM; Bunge, MB. Transplantation of Schwann cells and/or olfactory ensheathing glia into the contused spinal cord: Survival, migration, axon association, and functional recovery. *Glia.* 2007; 55: 976–1000.

[56] Bunge, MB. Novel combination strategies to repair the injured mammalian spinal cord. *J Spinal Cord Med.* 2008; 31: 262–9.

[57] Duncan, ID; Aguayo, AJ; Bunge, RP; Wood, PM. Transplantation of rat Schwann cells grown in tissue culture into the mouse spinal cord. *J Neurol Sci.* 1981;49:241-52

[58] Fouad, K; Schnell, L; Bunge, MB; Schwab, ME; Liebscher, T; Pearse, DD. Combining Schwann cell bridges and olfactory-ensheathing glia grafts with chondroitinase promotes locomotor recovery after complete transaction of the spinal cord. *J. Neurosci.* 25:1169–1178; 2005.

[59] Ramon-Cueto, A; Cordero, MI; Santos-Benito, FF; Avila, J. Functional recovery of paraplegic rats and motor axon regeneration in their spinal cords by olfactory ensheathing glia. *Neuron* 2000; 25:425–435.

[60] Li, Y; Field, PM; Raisman, G. Repair of adult rat corticospinal tract by transplants of olfactory ensheathing cells. *Science.* 1997;277:2000-2.

[61] García-Alias, G; Lopez-Vales, R; Fores, J; Navarro, X; Verdu, E. Acute transplantation of olfactory ensheathing cells or Schwann cells promotes recovery after spinal cord injury in the rat. *J. Neurosci. Res.* 2004; 75:632–641.

[62] Munoz-Quiles, C; Santos-Benito, FF; Llamusí, MB; Ramon-Cueto, A. Chronic spinal injury repair by olfactory bulb ensheathing glia and feasibility for autologous therapy. *J. Neuropathol. Exp. Neurol.* 2009;68:1294–1308.

[63] Kubasak, MD; Jindrich, DL; Zhong, H; Takeoka, A; McFarland, KC; Munoz-Quiles, C; Roy, RR; Edgerton, VR; Ramon-Cueto, A; Phelps, P. OEG implantation and step training enhance hindlimb-stepping ability in adult spinal transected rats. *Brain* 2008; 131:264–276.

[64] Imaizumi, T; Lankford, KL; Waxman, SG; Greer, CA; Kocsis, JD. Transplanted olfactory ensheathing cells remyelinate and enhance

axonal conduction in the demyelinated dorsal columns of the rat spinal cord. *J. Neurosci.* 1998;18:6176–6185.

[65] Ruitenberg, MJ; Levison, DB; Lee, SV; Verhaagen, J; Harvey, AR; Plant, GW. NT-3 expression from engineered olfactory ensheathing glia promotes spinal sparing and regeneration. *Brain* 2005;128:839–853.

[66] Barnett, SC; Alexander, CL; Iwashita, Y; Gilson, JM; Crowther, J; Clark, L; Dunn, LT; Papanastassiou, V; Kennedy, PG; Franklin, RJ. Identification of a human olfactory ensheathing cell that can effect transplant-mediated remyelination of demyelinated CNS axons. *Brain.* 2000;123:1581-1588.

[67] Kato, T; Honmou, O; Uede, T; Hashi, K; Kocsis, JD. Transplantation of human olfactory ensheathing cells elicits remyelination of demyelinated rat spinal cord. *Glia* 2000;30:209–218.

[68] Jeffery, ND; Crang, AJ; O'leary, MT; Hodge, SJ; Blakemore, WF. Behavioural consequences of oligodendrocyte progenitor cell transplantation into experimental demyelinating lesions in the rat spinal cord. *Eur J Neurosci* 1999, 11:1508–1514.

[69] Lee, KH, Yoon, DH, Park, YG, Lee, BH. Effects of glial transplantation on functional recovery following acute spinal cord injury. *J Neurotrauma* 2005, 22:575–589.

[70] Spilker, MH; Yannas, IV; Kostyk, SK; Norregaard, TV;Hsu, HP; Spector, M. The effects of tubulation on healing and scar formation after transection of the adult rat spinal cord. *Restor. Neurol. Neurosci.* 2001, 18, 23−28.

[71] King, VR; Alovskaya, A; Wei, DY; Brown, RA; Priestley, JV. The use of injectable forms of fibrin and fibronectin to support axonal ingrowth after spinal cord injury. *Biomaterials* 2010;31: 4447−4456.

[72] Li, X; Yang, Z; Zhang, A.; Wang, T; Chen, W. Repair of thoracic spinal cord injury by chitosan tube implantation in adult rats. *Biomaterials* 2009, 30, 1121−1132.

[73] Olson, HE; Rooney, GE; Gross, L; Nesbitt, JJ; Galvin, KE; Knight, A; Chen, B; Yaszemski, MJ; Windebank, AJ. Neural stem cell- and Schwann cell-loaded biodegradable polymer scaffolds support axonal regeneration in the transected spinal cord. *Tissue Eng. Part A* 2009, 15, 1797−1805.

[74] Teng, YD; Choi, H; Onario, RC; Zhu, S; Desilets, FC; Lan, S; Woodard, EJ; Snyder, EY; Eichler, ME; Friedlander, RM. Minocycline inhibits contusion-triggered mitochondrial cytochrome C release and mitigates

functional deficits after spinal cord injury. *Proc. Natl. Acad. Sci.* 2004, 101, 3071–3076.

[75] Nomura, H; Zahir, T; Kim, H; Katayama, Y; Kulbatski, I; Morshead, CM; Shoichet, MS; Tator, C H. Extramedullary chitosan channels promote survival of transplanted neural stem and progenitor cells and create a tissue bridge after complete spinal cord transection. *Tissue Eng. Part A* 2008,14, 649–665.

[76] Wang, JM; Zeng, YS; Wu, JL; Li, Y; Teng, YD. Cograft of neural stem cells and Schwann cells overexpressing TrkC and neurotrophin-3, respectively, after rat spinal cord transection. *Biomaterials* 2011, 32, 7454–7468.

[77] Nomura, H; Zahir, T; Kim, H; Katayama, Y; Kulbatski, I; Morshead, CM; Shoichet, MS; Tator, CH. Extramedullary chitosan channels promote survival of transplanted neural stem and progenitor cells and create a tissue bridge after complete spinal cord transection. *Tissue Eng Part A* 2008, 14:649–665.

[78] Johnson, PJ; Tatara, A; McCreedy, DA; Shiu, A; Sakiyama-Elbert, SE. Tissueengineered fibrin scaffolds containing neural progenitors enhance functional recovery in a subacute model of SCI. *Soft Matter* 2010, 6:5127–5137.

[79] Prakash, S; Soe-Lin, H. Strategy for cell therapy: polymers for live cell encapsulation and delivery. *Trends Biomater Artif Organs* 2004, 18:24–35.

[80] Borjigin, M; Strouse, B; Niamat, RA; Bialk, P; Eskridge, C; Xie, J; Kmiec, EB. Proliferation of genetically modified human cells on electrospun nanofiber scaffolds. *Mol Ther Nucleic Acids* 2012, 1, e59.

[81] Schnell, E; Klinkhammer, K; Balzer, S; Brook, G; Klee, D; Dalton, P; Mey, J. Guidance of glial cell migration and axonal growth on electrospun nanofibers of poly-epsilon-caprolactone and a collagen/poly-epsilon-caprolactone blend. *Biomaterials.* 2007,28, 3012–3025.

[82] Yao, L; O'Brien, N; Windebank, A; Pandit, A. Orienting neurite growth in electrospun fibrous neural conduits. *J. Biomed. Mater. Res. B Appl. Biomater.* 2009, 90, 483–491.

[83] Zander, NE; Orlicki, JA; Rawlett, AM; Beebe, TP, Jr. Surface-modified nanofibrous biomaterial bridge for the enhancement and control of neurite outgrowth. *Biointerphases* 2010, 5, 149–158.

[84] Prabhakaran, MP; Venugopal, JR; Chyan, TT; Hai, LB; Chan, CK; Lim, AY; Ramakrishna, S. Electrospun biocomposite nanofibrous scaffolds for neural tissue engineering. *Tissue Eng. Part A*. 2008, 14, 1787–1797.

[85] Zamani, F; Amani-Tehran, M; Latifi, M; Shokrgozar, MA; Zaminy, A. Promotion of spinal cord axon regeneration by 3D nanofibrous core-sheath scaffolds. *J. Biomed. Mater. Res.* A 2013.

[86] Wang, W; Itoh, S; Konno, K; Kikkawa, T; Ichinose, S; Sakai, K; Ohkuma, T; Watabe, K. Effects of Schwann cell alignment along the oriented electrospun chitosan nanofibers on nerve regeneration. *J. Biomed. Mater. Res.* A 2009, 91, 994–1005.

[87] Neal, RA; Tholpady, SS; Foley, PL; Swami, N; Ogle, RC; Botchwey, EA. Alignment and composition of laminin-polycaprolactone nanofiber blends enhance peripheral nerve regeneration. *J. Biomed. Mater. Res. A* 2011, 100, 406–423.

[88] Yu, W; Zhao, W; Zhu, C; Zhang, X; Ye, D; Zhang, W; Zhou, Y; Jiang, X; Zhang, Z. Sciatic nerve regeneration in rats by a promising electrospun collagen/poly(ε-caprolactone) nerve conduit with tailored degradation rate. *BMC Neurosci.* 2011, 12, 68.

[89] Weightman, A; Jenkins, S; Pickard, M; Chari, D; Yang Y. Alignment of multiple glial cell populations in 3D nanofiber scaffolds: toward the development of multicellular implantable scaffolds for repair of neural injury. Nanomedicine. 2014, 10, 291-295.

[90] Ranjan, OP; Shavi, GV; Nayak, UY; Arumugam, K; Averineni, RK; Meka, SR; Sureshwar, P. Controlled release chitosan microspheres of mirtazapine: in vitro and in vivo evaluation. *Arch Pharm Res* 2011, 34:1919–1929.

[91] Zhao, Q; Han B; Wang, Z; Gao, C; Peng, C; Shen, J. Hollow chitosan-alginate multilayer microcapsules as drug delivery vehicle:doxorubicin loading and in vitro and in vivo studies. *Nanomedicine* 2007, 3:63–74.

[92] Mathew, ST; Devi, SG; Prasanth, VV; Vinod, B. Formulation and in vitro-in vivo evaluation of ketoprofen-loaded albumin microspheres for intramuscular administration. *J Microencapsul* 2009, 26:456–469.

[93] Yao, R; Zhang, R; Luan, J, Lin F. Alginate and alginate/gelatin microspheres for human adipose-derived stem cell encapsulation and differentiation. *Biofabrication* 2012, 4:025007.

[94] Chan, BP; Hui, TY; Wong, MY; Yip, KH; Chan, GC. Mesenchymal stem cell encapsulated collagen microspheres for bone tissue engineering. *Tissue Eng Part C Methods* 2010, 16:225–235.

[95] Yao, L; Phan, F; Li, Y. Collagen microsphere serving as a cell carrier supports oligodendrocyte progenitor cell growth and differentiation for neurite myelination in vitro. *Stem Cell Res Ther*. 2013, 4, 109.

[96] Cao, Q; Xu, XM; Devries, WH; Enzmann, GU; Ping, P; Tsoulfas, P; Wood, PM; Bunge, MB; Whittemore, SR. Functional recovery in traumatic spinal cord injury after transplantation of multineurotrophin-expressing glial-restricted precursor cells. *J Neurosci.* 2005;25:6947-57.

[97] Chau, CH; Shum, DK, Li; H, Pei, J; Lui, YY; Wirthlin, L; Chan, YS; Xu, XM. Chondroitinase ABC enhances axonal regrowth through Schwann cell-seeded guidance channels after spinal cord injury. *FASEB J.* 2004;18:194-6.

[98] Xu, XM; Chen, A; Guénard, V; Kleitman, N; Bunge, MB. Bridging Schwann cell transplants promote axonal regeneration from both the rostral and caudal stumps of transected adult rat spinal cord. *J. Neurocytol.* 26:1–16; 1997.

[99] Xu, X. M.; Guénard, V.; Kleitman, M.; Bunge, M. B. Axonal regeneration into Schwann cell-seeded guidance channels grafted into transected adult rat spinal cord. *J. Comp. Neurol.* 35:145–160; 1995.

[100] Williams, RR; Henao, M; Pearse, DD; Bunge, MB. Permissive Schwann cell graft/spinal cord interfaces for axon regeneration. *Cell Transplant.* 2015;24:115-31.

[101] Richardson, PM; McGuinness, UM; Aguayo, AJ. Peripheral nerve autografts to the rat spinal cord: Studies with axonal tracing methods. *Brain Res.* 237:147–162; 1982.

[102] Chan, JR; Watkins, TA; Cosgaya, JM; Zhang, C; Chen, L;Reichardt, LF; Shooter, EM; Barres, BA. NGF controls axonal receptivity to myelination by Schwann cells or oligodendrocytes. *Neuron.* 2004, 43, 183−191.

[103] Wang, H; Tewari, A; Einheber, S; Salzer, JL; Melendez-Vasquez, CV. Myosin II has distinct functions in PNS and CNS myelin sheath formation. *J. Cell Biol.* 2008, 182, 1171−1184.

[104] O'Meara, RW; Ryan, SD; Colognato, H; Kothary, R. Derivation of enriched oligodendrocyte cultures and oligodendrocyte/neuron myelinating co-cultures from post-natal murine tissues. *J. Vis. Exp.* 2011, 54, pii:3324.

[105] Lee, S; Chong, SY; Tuck, SJ; Corey, JM; Chan, JR. A rapid and reproducible assay for modeling myelination by oligodendrocytes using engineered nanofibers. *Nat. Protoc.* 2013, 8, 771−782.

[106] Li, Y; Ceylan, M; Shrestha, B; Wang, H; Lu, QR; Asmatulu, R; Yao, L. Nanofibers support oligodendrocyte precursor cell growth and function as a neuron-free model for myelination study. *Biomacromolecules.* 2014, 15, 319-326.

[107] Fawcett, JW; Curt, A; Steeves, JD; Coleman, WP; Tuszynski, MH; Lammertse, D; Bartlett, PF; Blight, AR; Dietz, V; Ditunno, J; Dobkin, BH; Havton, LA; Ellaway, PH; Fehlings, MG; Privat, A; Grossman, R; Guest, JD; Kleitman, N; Nakamura, M; Gaviria, M; Short, D. Guidelines for the conduct of clinical trials for spinal cord injury as developed by the ICCP panel: spontaneous recovery after spinal cord injury and statistical power needed for therapeutic clinical trials. *Spinal Cord.* 2007; 45:190 –205.

[108] Lammertse, D; Tuszynski, MH; Steeves, JD; Curt, A; Fawcett, JW; Rask, C; Ditunno, JF; Fehlings, MG; Guest, JD; Ellaway, PH; Kleitman, N; Blight, AR; Dobkin, BH; Grossman, R; Katoh, H; Privat, A; Kalichman, M. Guidelines for the conduct of clinical trials for spinal cord injury as developed by the ICCP panel: clinical trial design. *Spinal Cord.* 2007; 45:232–242.

[109] Steeves, JD; Lammertse, D; Curt, A; Fawcett, JW; Tuszynski, MH; Ditunno, JF; Ellaway, PH; Fehlings, MG; Guest, JD; Kleitman, N; Bartlett, PF; Blight, AR; Dietz, V; Dobkin, BH; Grossman, R; Short, D; Nakamura, M; Coleman, WP; Gaviria, M; Privat, A. Guidelines for the conduct of clinical trials for spinal cord injury (SCI) as developed by the ICCP panel: clinical trial outcome measures. *Spinal Cord.* 2007; 45:206 –221.

[110] Tuszynski, MH; Steeves, JD; Fawcett, JW; Lammertse, D; Kalichman, M; Rask, C; Curt, A; Ditunno, JF; Fehlings, MG; Guest, JD; Ellaway, PH; Kleitman, N; Bartlett, PF; Blight, AR; Dietz, V; Dobkin, BH; Grossman, R; Privat, A. Guidelines for the conduct of clinical trials for spinal cord injury as developed by the ICCP panel: clinical trial inclusion/exclusion criteria and ethics. *Spinal Cord.* 2007;45:222–231.

[111] Mackay-Sim, A; Féron, F; Cochrane, J; Bassingthwaighte, L; Bayliss, C; Davies, W; Fronek, P; Gray, C; Kerr, G; Licina, P; Nowitzke, A; Perry, C; Silburn, PA; Urquhart, S; Geraghty, T. Autologous olfactory ensheathing cell transplantation in human paraplegia: a 3-year clinical trial. *Brain.* 2008;131:2376-86.

[112] Lima, C; Pratas-Vital, J; Escada, P; Hasse-Ferreira, A; Capucho, C; Peduzzi, JD. Olfactory mucosa autografts in human spinal cord injury: a pilot clinical study. *J Spinal Cord Med.* 2006;29:191-203; discussion 204-6.

[113] Chhabra HS, Lima C, Sachdeva S, Mittal A, Nigam V, Chaturvedi D, Arora M, Aggarwal A, Kapur R, Khan TA. Autologous olfactory

[corrected] mucosal transplant in chronic spinal cord injury: an Indian *Pilot Study. Spinal Cord.* 20

[114] Huang H, Wang H, Chen L, Gu Z, Zhang J, Zhang F, Song Y, Li Y, Tan K, Liu Y, Xi H. Influence factors for functional improvement after olfactory ensheathing cell transplantation for chronic spinal cord injury. *Zhongguo Xiu Fu Chong Jian Wai Ke Za Zhi.* 2006;20:434-8.

[115] Lima C, Escada P, Pratas-Vital J, Branco C, Arcangeli CA, Lazzeri G, Maia CA, Capucho C, Hasse-Ferreira A, Peduzzi JD. Olfactory mucosal autografts and rehabilitation for chronic traumatic spinal cord injury. *Neurorehabil Neural Repair*. 2010 Jan;24(1):10-22.

[116] Dobkin BH, Curt A, Guest J. Cellular transplants in China: observational study from the largest human experiment in chronic spinal cord injury. *Neurorehabil Neural Repair*. 2006; 20:5-13.

[117] Bunge, RP. Changing use of nerve tissue culture 1950–1975. In: Tower, D. B., ed. The nervous system, volume one: The basic neurosciences. New York, NY: *Raven Press;* 1975:31–42.

[118] Saberi H, Moshayedi P, Aghayan HR, Arjmand B, Hosseini SK, Emami-Razavi SH, Rahimi-Movaghar V, Raza M, Firouzi M. Treatment of chronic thoracic spinal cord injury patients with autologous Schwann cell transplantation: an interim report on safety considerations and possible outcomes. *Neurosci Lett*. 2008;443:46-50.

In: Oligodendrocytes
Editor: Dana Swanson

ISBN: 978-1-63483-330-1

Chapter 4

Oligodendrocyte Plasticity: Role of Growth Factors and Axon Proteins during Demyelination and Remyelination

Catherine Fressinaud[*,†]
LUNAM, Neurology Department, University Hospital, Angers Cedex, France
LUNAM, Neurobiology and Transgenesis Laboratory, University Hospital, Angers Cedex, France

Abstract

Oligodendrocytes (OL) are the main target of the pathological process during Multiple Sclerosis (MS). OL death and demyelination are constantly observed in MS lesions, together with axon damage and decrease in axon cytoskeleton protein (neurofilaments, tubulin) expression. Remyelination may occur but is never complete, leading to permanent disability. Mature myelinating OL are the main cells of the OL lineage in the adult central nervous system (CNS) and may participate,

[*] Correspondence to: Dr Catherine Fressinaud, MD, PhD, Neurology Department, University Hospital, 4 rue Larrey, 49933 Angers Cedex 9, France. E-mail: catherine.fressinaud@univ-angers.fr. Phone: 33 (0)2 44 68 84 92. Fax: 33 (0)2 41 35 35 94.

together with OL progenitors (OLP) in lesion repair. However the capacity of these cells to survive insults, to grow new processes, and to synthesize new myelin sheaths is partly unknown. The molecules driving this phenomenon have not been deciphered yet. We review some of our data showing the induction of some plasticity of OL by growth factors and axon proteins *in vitro*. Restricted plasticity also was observed *in vivo*, in murine demyelinating lesions, and in MS lesions.

Despite the fact that mature myelinating OL represent the ultimate differentiation stage of OL development, *in vitro* some growth factors such as basic fibroblast growth factor (bFGF) are able to induce partial dedifferentiation of the cells with decreased myelin basic protein (MBP) expression and synthesis of loose myelin membranes (Fressinaud et al., 1995). Using lysophosphatidyl choline (LPC) as a toxic demyelinating agent, it was also observed that either bFGF or platelet-derived growth factor (PDGF) increase OL survival and synthesis of new myelin membranes *in vitro*. Similarly unique demyelinating events in rat demyelinating paradigm result in complete remyelination, and single stereotactic injection of growth factors (PDGF, neurotrophin-3 (NT-3)) accelerate this repair (Allamargot et al., 2001; Jean et al., 2003). However MS often occurs in a remittent-relapsing course and remyelination fails. The capacity of OL to survive multiple insults was demonstrated to be diminished *in vitro* with our LPC model, even in the presence of growth factors (Fressinaud, 2005). This was akin to analysis of OL and myelinated fibers in MS lesions compared to the adjacent normal appearing white matter (Fressinaud, 2007). As could be expected the number of OL was decreased in MS lesions, moreover the number of myelinated fibers per cell was decreased even more. Similar results were obtained with LPC lesions *in vivo* since controls (incomplete remyelination) showed a lower number of myelinated fibers per OL than NT-3-treated animals (robust remyelination).

Axons, which undergo degenerative changes during demyelination, are one of the main partners of OL; however, their crosstalk is poorly identified. We have shown that, following LPC and PDGF injection, remyelination alleviates these axonal lesions with an increase in NF expression in the rat model. Nevertheless, a striking event during MS is the release of NF and tubulin (TUB) in the cerebrospinal fluid, probably as a result of axon lesions. However, the role of NF when they are outside from the axon was unknown. We observed that NF, and other cytoskeleton proteins from the axon, as well as synthetic peptides corresponding to specific NF sequences increase OL growth, and differentiation. In addition, these proteins and peptides increase OL survival and partially protect them from LPC toxicity *in vitro*. Thus, these proteins could participate *in vivo* in a subtle bidirectional crosstalk with OL. Thus, extracellular NF could favorize OL plasticity and myelin repair, whereas in return remyelination could promote axon regeneration.

Keywords: astrocyte, axon-glia interactions, demyelination; microtubule, neurofilament

Abbreviations

Ab	antibody;
ARA-C	cytosine arabinoside;
AS	astrocytes;
bFGF	basic fibroblast growth factor;
BrdU	bromodeoxyuridine;
CDM	chemically-defined medium;
CNP	2', 3'-cyclic nucleotide 3'-phosphodiesterase;
CNS	central nervous system;
CONT	control;
CSF	cerebrospinal fluid;
EAE	experimental autoimmune encephalitis;
GFAP	glial fibrillary acidic protein;
LPC	lysophosphatidyl choline;
mAb	monoclonal antibody;
MAPs	microtubule associated proteins;
MBP	myelin basic protein;
MOG	myelin oligodendrocyte protein;
MS	multiple sclerosis;
NF	neurofilaments;
NT-3	neurotrophin-3;
OL	oligodendrocyte;
OLP	oligodendrocyte progenitor;
PDGF	platelet-derived growth factor;
PLP	proteolipid protein;
SCR	scrambled;
SpbII	spectrin β2;
SYN2	synapsin II;
TBS	tubulin-binding site;
TEM	transmission electron microscopy;
TUB	tubulin.

Introduction

Oligodendrocytes (OL) are the main target of the pathological process during Multiple Sclerosis (MS). OL death and demyelination are constantly observed in lesions, together with axon damage and a decrease in the expression of main axon cytoskeleton proteins (i.e., neurofilaments, and tubulin).

Remyelination may occur but is never complete, leading to permanent disability in patients. Mature myelinating OL are the main cells of the OL lineage in the adult central nervous system (CNS) and could participate, together with OL progenitors (OLP) in lesion repair. However the capacity of these cells to survive insults, to grow new processes, and to synthesize new myelin sheaths is partly unknown. The molecules driving this phenomenon have not been deciphered yet. We review some of our data showing the induction of some plasticity of OL by growth factors and axon proteins *in vitro*. Experimentally, some plasticity is also observed *in vivo* in demyelinating lesions induced by lysophosphatidyl choline (LPC), and is upregulated by growth factors. On the contrary, we have observed in MS lesions that OL plasticity is decreased. In the light of our results we suggest several hypotheses about the involvement of OL plasticity in remyelination during MS.

Growth Factors Induce OL Plasticity *In Vitro*

Part of our study was conducted in newborn rat secondary OL cultures (Fressinaud et al., 1990; 1993). These cultures are grown in chemically-defined medium (CDM). They are at least 95% pure, and contain both OL progenitors (OLP), characterized by A2B5 monoclonal antibody (mAb), as well as differentiated OL labeled by anti-2',3'-cyclic nucleotide 3'-phosphodiesterase (CNP+) mAb, and mature OL expressing myelin basic protein (MBP) (Figure 1). Under basal conditions around 20% OLP proliferate as determined by bromodeoxyuridine (BrdU) incorporation and immunostaining of the nuclei with anti-BrdU mAb. On the contrary CNP+ and MBP + OL are post mitotic cells. Despite the lack of neurons in these cultures MBP + OL synthesize myelin-like membranes with morphological and biochemical characteristics very similar to myelin *in vivo* (Figure 1) (Fressinaud et al., 1990).

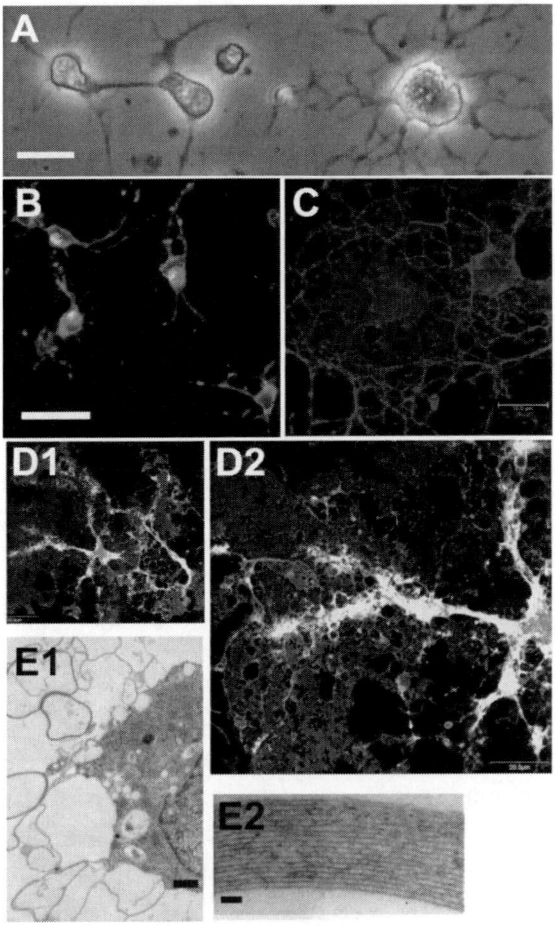

Figure 1. Characterization of oligodendrocyte cultures. (A) OL progenitors (left) differentiate into mature OL (right) characterized by multiple ramified processes, phase contrast microscopy; bar = 20 μm. (B) OL progenitors are labeled by A2B5 antibody (green), their proliferation is evidenced by nuclear immunostaining for bromodeoxyuridine (red), merger of Alexa 488 and Alexa 568 fields; bar = 20 μm. (C) Differentiated OL with complex mutibranched processes are labeled by anti-CNP Ab (red), nuclei stain: Hoechst, bar = 10 μm. (D) Mature OL exhibit very complex processes and myelin-like membranes, double immunolabeling for MBP (green) and CNP (red), myelin-like enwrapments can be observed at higher magnification in (D2), confocal microscopy, merger of fields; bar = 50 μm in D1, 20 μm in D2. (E) Transmission electron microscopy demonstrating numerous myelin balls attached to the cell body of an OL (E1), at higher magnification (E2) these enwrapments correspond to myelin-like structures with major and minor dense lines, and membrane compaction identical to what is observed *in vitro* (≈ 14 nm); bar = 500 nm in E1, 50 nm in E2.

Growth Factors Improve Myelin Synthesis *In Vitro* after a Chemical Attack

Therefore, this paradigm was useful in testing the effects of demyelinating agents such as lysophosphatidyl choline (LPC) (Waxmann et al., 1979), and to determine whether some growth factors could improve remyelination. Addition of LPC (24 h, 2.10^{-5} M) induced 50% cell death. Both OLP and mature OL died, and transmission electron microscopy (TEM) revealed the disappearance of myelin-like membranes (Figure 2). Spontaneous recovery in CDM was tenuous, with the apparent survival of some cells, but proliferation was decreased by 65%, and regeneration of cell processes and myelin-like membranes was scarce. Immunocytochemical studies with A2B5 mAb, and anti-MBP polyclonal Ab showed that the entire OL lineage was affected by LPC at all stages of maturation. On the contrary, proliferation, differentiation, and myelin-like membrane synthesis were partly restored by growth factors such as basic fibroblast growth factor (bFGF) (10 ng/mL) (Figure 2). A 3 day treatment with bFGF induced the reconstruction of myelin-like membranes, albeit less compacted than in untreated controls. The doubling in the number of cells and the 46% increase in proliferation was essentially due to the proliferation of OLP. Similar results were obtained with platelet derived growth factor (PDGF) (15 ng/mL), or neurotrophin-3 (NT-3) (5 ng/mL) (not shown).

Thus, after one injury growth factors induced OL plasticity as evidenced by upregulation of OLP proliferation, and of the ability of mature OL to regrow processes and synthesize new myelin-like membranes *in vitro* (Fressinaud and Vallat, 1994).

bFGF Induces Mature OL Dedifferentiation and Decompaction of Myelin-like Membranes

To characterize further these effects of growth factors we tested them in cultures enriched in mature OL. To obtain homogeneous cultures of mature OL, cells were treated with cytosine arabinoside (ARA-C) which kills OLP that proliferate (Fressinaud et al., 1992). OL cultures were either grown in CDM alone (control), or treated with 10^{-5} M cytosine arabinoside (ARA-C) for the first 3 days. On the third day, the ARA-C-treated cells were washed twice, and the cells were grown in fresh CDM alone, or treated daily with 10 ng/mL bovine bFGF from the third to the sixth day of the secondary culture. In order to assess the reversibility of the bFGF effects, cell cultures treated as described above with ARA-C and bFGF were washed twice with CDM on the sixth day and grown further in CDM alone until the 9th or the 12th day.

In cultures treated with ARA-C and bFGF numerous myelin-like membranes were observable, nevertheless the periodicity of the enwrapments was irregular and the period increased over 18 nm and up to 24 nm, contrary to the compacted sheaths observed in controls and ARA-C treated cells (Figure 3). This was associated with a decrease in OL expressing maturation features observed by immunocytochemistry: the expression of MBP, and of other myelin proteins such as proteolipid (PLP), and myelin oligodendrocyte glycoprotein (MOG) was reduced. Moreover, cell morphology returned to immature OL phenotype with fewer processes that were poorly branched (Figure 3) (Fressinaud et al., 1995).

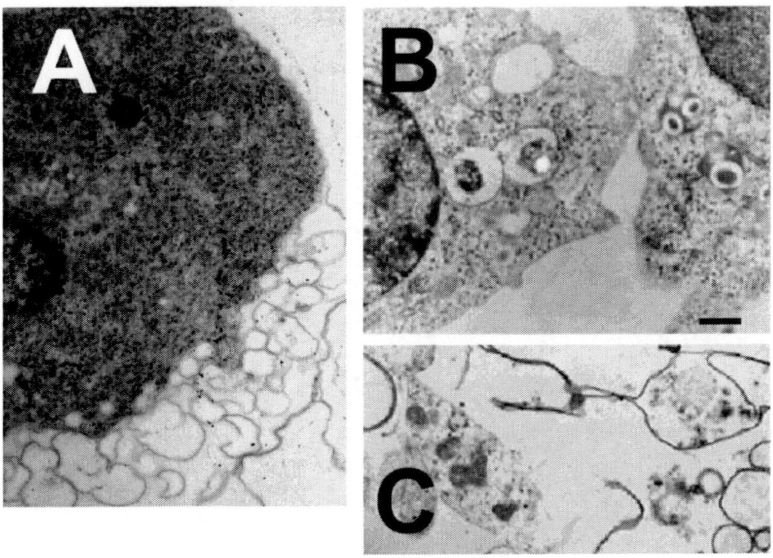

Figure 2. Transmission electron microscopy demonstrating numerous myelin balls attached to the cell body of an OL in control cultures (A); these membranes are destroyed by LPC (B). On the contrary new myelin-like enwrapments are synthesized when bFGF treatment is added to cultures for 3 days after LPC (C); bar = 500 nm.

These results contrast with previous descriptions of mature OL as post-mitotic cells, fixed at the final stage of OL differentiation. They demonstrate another facet of plasticity induced by growth factors *in vitro*: i.e., mature OL are able to dedifferentiate, at least partly, in the presence of some growth factors.

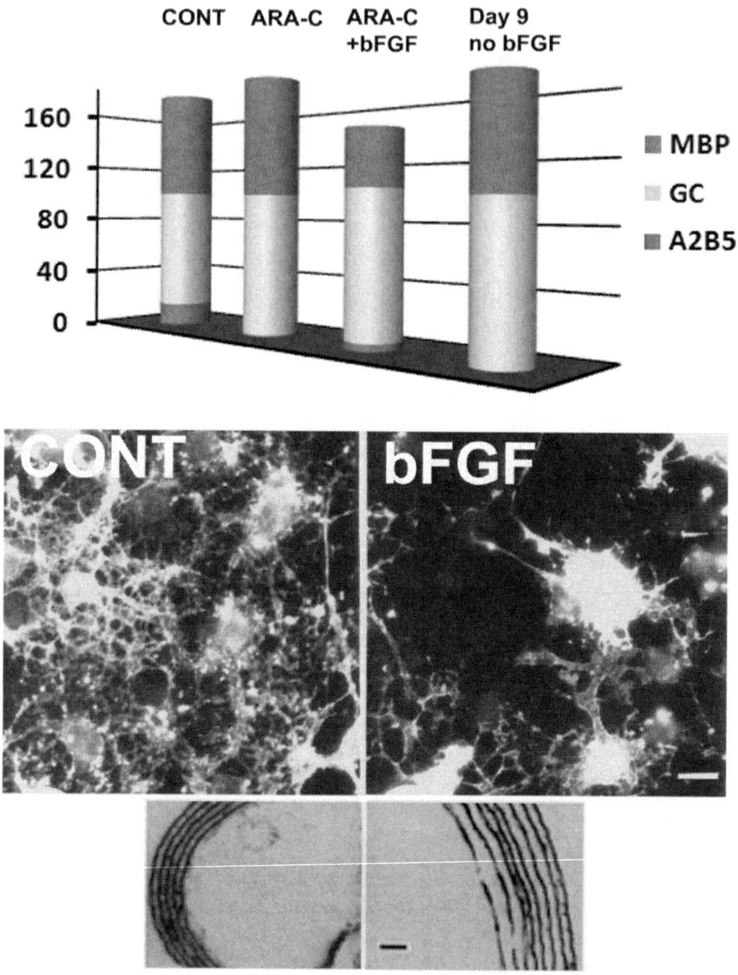

Figure 3. Chronic treatment of OL cultures with bFGF induces mature OL to dedifferentiate. Graph showing the decrease in percentage of MBP+ OL in cultures treated daily with bFGF (ARA-C + bFGF), on day 6, compared to control (CONT) and to cytosine arabinoside treated cultures (ARA-C + bFGF). When bFGF is removed for the following 3 days, the percentage of MBP + OL increases to previous levels (no bFGF, day 9). Immunocytochemistry for MBP (optic microscopy) shows a decrease in MBP immunostaining in bFGF treated cells compared to controls; bar = 20 μm. Loss of MBP is also evidenced by TEM demonstrating uncompacted myelin-like membranes in bFGF treated OL (right) compared to controls (left); bar = 50 nm.

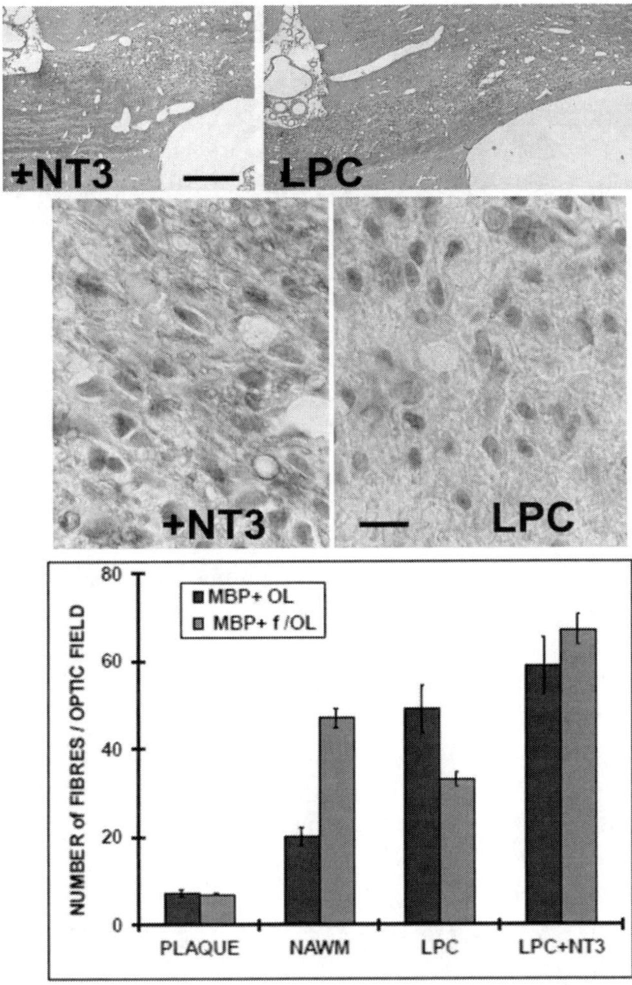

Figure 4. Neurotrophin-3 improves remyelination *in vivo*. Fifteen days after LPC stereotactic microinjection into rat corpus callosum, the demyelinated area (characterized by loss of luxol blue staining: pink colored) is strongly reduced in NT-3 treated animals (left) versus LPC only (right), luxol and hematein counterstain (upper panels); bar = 100 μm. This is also demonstrated by MBP immunostaining in the center of the lesion, showing numerous myelinated fibers in NT-3 treated animals versus LPC; MBP immunostaining revealed by peroxidase, hematein counterstain (middle panels); bar = 20 μm. OL capacity to synthesize myelin during remyelination (number of myelinated fibers per OL, blue bars) is compared in MS between lesion (plaque) and normal appearing white matter (NAWM), and in the center of the lesion between LPC induced lesion versus LPC + NT-3 treated animals. This demonstrates that in both conditions demyelination affects even more the capacity of each cell to synthesize myelin, than the number of OL per se (black bars).

OL Plasticity Induced by Growth Factors *In Vivo*

Induction of OLP proliferation as well as improvement of recovery after LPC treatment by bFGF, PDGF (Fressinaud et al., 1996), or NT-3 suggested that they could promote remyelination *in vivo*. This was demonstrated in demyelinating lesions induced by stereotactic microinjection of 1% LPC (1 μL) in the corpus callosum of adult rats. Growth factors were injected 0.02 mm above LPC and at the same time. LPC induced demyelination is easily observable on luxol stained sections (Figure 4); spontaneous recovery is complete in one month. After 15 days, in animals treated with PDGF (1 μg) or NT-3 (1 μg) the volume of the demyelinated area was significantly reduced (by 56%) compared to untreated controls (LPC alone) (Allamargot et al., 2001; Jean et al., 2003). Similarly, the number of cells of the OL lineage was upregulated, and immunohistochemistry showed an increase in mature MBP+ OL number (+ 66%) in treated animals. The number of fibers immunostained for MBP was also increased by PDGF or NT-3 (Figure 4). Improvement of remyelination was confirmed by TEM: there were more myelinated fibers and thicker myelin sheaths than in controls (not shown) (Allamargot et al., 2001; Jean et al., 2003). Since less than 3% axons degenerate in this model, and as the astrocytic gliosis was not modified, these data indicate that PDGF and NT-3 act directly on cells of the OL lineage to enhance their plasticity, and promote remyelination *in vivo,* as could be expected.

OL Plasticity Is Restricted After Multiple Insults *In Vitro*

Strikingly, even in the absence of growth factor treatment, single lesions like those induced by LPC completely remyelinate spontaneously as discussed above. On the contrary, in MS relapses occur and remyelination fails. It has been hypothesized that this results from OL and/or OLP loss as a consequence of repeated attacks (e.g., Rodriguez et al., 1993; Ozawa et al., 1994; Mews et al., 1998; Wolswijk, 2000; Brück et al., 1994, 2002; Chang et al., 2002). Nevertheless, Penderis et al., (2003) reported that two to three episodes of ethidium bromide-induced demyelination did not result in OLP depletion in the rat CNS when intervening recovery was allowed. In contrast, Mason et al.,

(2004) observed the depletion of OL and OLP in a similar model. Other groups (e.g., Chang et al., 2002) have described quite numerous OL contacting axons, though without proper differentiation or remyelination in MS lesions. Based on these contradictory reports we tested the hypothesis that some OL may survive a single insult, but that the recurrence of insults – as observed in MS - could be a limiting factor for repair. This study was performed *in vitro* by comparing OL survival after multiple versus single LPC treatments.

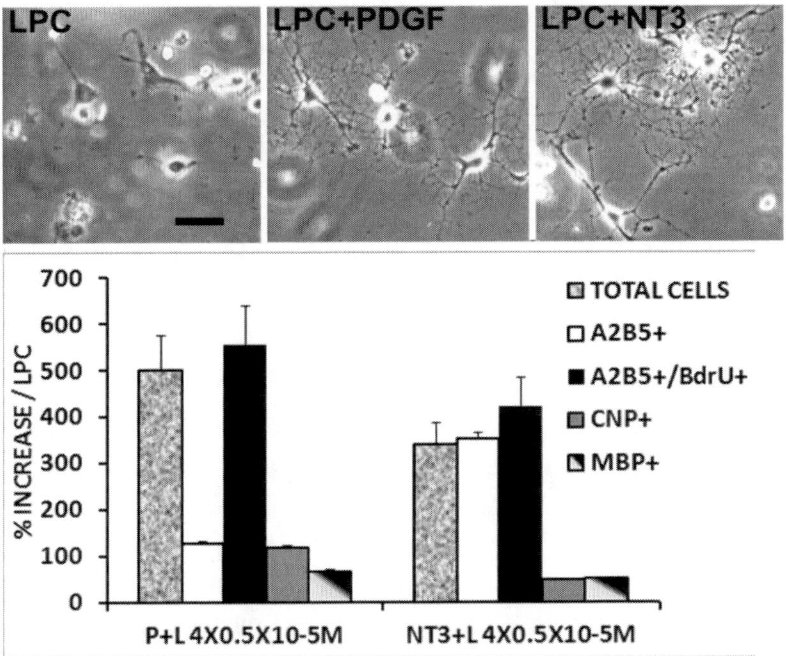

Figure 5. PDGF and NT-3 partly restore OL plasticity. After multiple treatments with LPC (LPC 4 X 0.5 X 10^{-5}M) OL death is pronounced, and surviving OL show a less differentiated morphology compared to controls (left). Despite LPC attacks PDGF or NT-3 treatment allows more cells to survive, and OL to extend more ramified processes (middle and right panels); phase contrast microscopy; bar = 20 μm. This is confirmed by immunocytochemistry showing a pronounced increase in total cells, as well as in proliferating OLP (A2B5+ cells), and mature OL (MBP+ cells) in PDGF treated cultures (P + L) as well as in NT-3 treated ones (NT3 + L). Results expressed as percentage of increase compared to cultures treated 4 times with LPC only, all differences are significant ($p < 0.01$).

Two types of insults were analyzed in OL cultures (see above): a unique treatment of 24 h with 2.10^{-5} M LPC (high concentration), versus multiple treatments, i.e., 4 treatments of 6 h each at low concentration (0.5 x 10^{-5} M). Thus, LPC was added for the same duration in total, although at ¼ concentration during multiple treatments. Between LPC treatments cells were grown in CDM alone, or supplemented with PDGF (15 ng/mL), or NT-3 (5 ng/mL) (Figure 5). Indeed, LPC added at low concentration to cultures for 4 short periods ($4^{*}6$ h) of time had a far more pronounced effect on OL death than a single treatment. Partial recovery was obtained by PDGF or NT-3 (Figure 5) with more than a 300% increase in total cell number after 6 days, compared to LPC alone. This corresponded mainly to OLP proliferation since differentiated (CNP +) and mature (MBP+) OL increased by less than 100% compared to LPC alone. Nevertheless, recovery induced by these growth factors did not reach the same extent as after a single LPC attack. Thus, *in vitro* the repetition of insults appeared to be an important phenomenon in the paucity of OL plasticity and regeneration (Fressinaud, 2005). This suggested that relapses in MS could similarly be involved in OL death and remyelination failure.

OL Plasticity and Remyelination *In Vivo*: Comparison of Animal Models with MS Lesions

To get further insight into these processes we had the opportunity to compare efficient remyelination (animals treated with growth factors after LPC induced demyelination, see above) on one side, and deficient remyelination (MS lesions) on the other. So, comparative analyses were performed between: i) LPC lesions in rat corpus callosum, versus LPC lesions in rat treated with NT-3 (15 days after injection, n = 18), and ii) MS lesions obtained from autopsies of 6 patients with secondary progressive chronic disease, versus adjacent normal-appearing white matter (NAWM) (18 samples) (Fressinaud, 2007).

In NT-3 treated animals, 15 days after LPC lesion, the number of MBP + OL had increased by 20% compared to untreated animals (LPC only) (Figure 4). In addition, the ratio of myelinated fibers per MBP + OL had increased by 100% compared to controls ($p < 0.05$). Similar results were obtained in PDGF treated animals (not shown) (Fressinaud, 2007). Thus it appeared that growth factor improvement of remyelination resulted from plasticity at the same time on the quantitative plan (increase in the number of OL) and qualitative plan (increase in myelinated internodes per OL).

Finally, in MS we also observed that OL had greatly decreased (40%) in most of the plaques (Figure 4), and that the number of myelinated (i.e., labeled with anti- MBP Ab) fibers per mature (MBP +) OL was constantly decreased (30-100%) in plaques compared with the NAWM. The reduction in the myelinating capacity of OL was considerable, on average there were 6.7 myelinated fibers per OL in plaques versus 47 in the NAWM.

This finding suggests that residual OL have a decreased ability to synthesize new myelin sheaths in MS, and that on the contrary OL capability to remyelinate axons is increased experimentally by growth factors. This defect in MS might result from exhaustion of OL after several relapses, in the light of our observations comparing multiple versus unique LPC insults *in vitro*.

Crosstalk: Interactions between OL and Axon Cytoskeleton Proteins during Demyelination/Remyelination

Axons undergo degenerative changes during demyelination, especially during MS (e.g., Trapp et al., 1998; Bitsch et al., 2000; De Luca et al., 2006; Defaux et al., 2010). They are the main partners of OL however their crosstalk is poorly identified. During MS, decreased expression of the main axon cytoskeleton proteins such as neurofilaments (NF) and tubulin (TUB) (Hoffman and Cleveland, 1988) has been observed in the demyelinated lesions by several groups (e.g., Trapp et al., 1998; Fressinaud et al., 2005). Experimentally we have shown also that, following LPC and PDGF injection, remyelination alleviates these axonal lesions with an increase in NF expression *in vivo* (Jean et al., 2002). Finally, it was reported that prompt axon remyelination protects from axonal loss, and that remyelination failure contributes to the axon loss that occurs in MS (Irvine and Blakemore, 2008). Nevertheless, whether demyelinated axons, expressing decreased levels of cytoskeleton proteins could, in turn, alter the remyelination process (as invaluable targets for remyelination) is unknown (Fressinaud and Sazdovitch, 2007).

In addition, a striking event during MS is the release of NF and TUB in the cerebrospinal fluid (CSF) (Lycke et al., 1998; Teunissen et al., 2005), where their concentration correlates with disease severity (relapse rate and disability) (Gresle et al., 2011; Kuhle et al., 2011; Schirmer et al., 2011). This probably occurs as a result of axon lesions. However, the mechanisms by which NF are released into the CSF during the evolution of MS are poorly documented, as well as their functions when they are present outside the axonal compartment. Reports on this subject indicate that experimentally NF are susceptible to proteolysis (Hall and Lee, 2005; Saatman et al., 2003), and NF light chain (NFL) positive macrophages have been identified in MS lesions (Huizinga et al., 2012).

Given the correlations previously established between myelin and axon alterations we have explored the role of axon cytoskeleton proteins in axon-OL interactions. We hypothesized that although these proteins are physiologically intracellular, they could become available for OL after release in the CSF during MS relapses. To determine whether proteins such as NF or TUB could exert a regulatory effect on OL during MS, pure OL cultures (see above) were used. Cytoskeleton proteins were first tested under basal conditions in CDM (Fressinaud et al., 2012). Then, to mimic demyelinating conditions, NF and TUB were assayed in cultures submitted to LPC (e.g., Fressinaud, 2005), to determine if they could regulate the repair process (Fressinaud and Eyer, 2013). NF were purified from rat brain by successive centrifugations as previously described (Fasani et al., 2004). The second pellet (NFP2) contains substantial amounts of TUB, whereas the fifth pellet (NFP5) is highly enriched in NF (Figure 6). Other purified axon cytoskeleton proteins were purchased as specified, and proteins from skin and liver also were used as controls (i.e., irrelevant proteins).

NF Purified Fractions Upregulate OL Proliferation and Maturation *In Vitro*

Depending on the purification step from which they were recovered, NF fractions either increased significantly OLP proliferation (NFP2, 2nd pellet), or their differentiation and maturation (NFP5, 5th pellet) (Figure 6) (Fressinaud et al., 2012). The concentration of 0.2μg/mL was found to have the maximal effect on OL cultures, and was used thereafter.

NFP2 fractions increased the total number of cells by 40% ($p < 0.01$, Student's t test). Immunolabeling confirmed that OLP cells have been induced to proliferate, since the relative percentage of A2B5 + /BrdU + cells increased by more than 120% versus controls ($p < 0.01$) (Figure 6C-D).

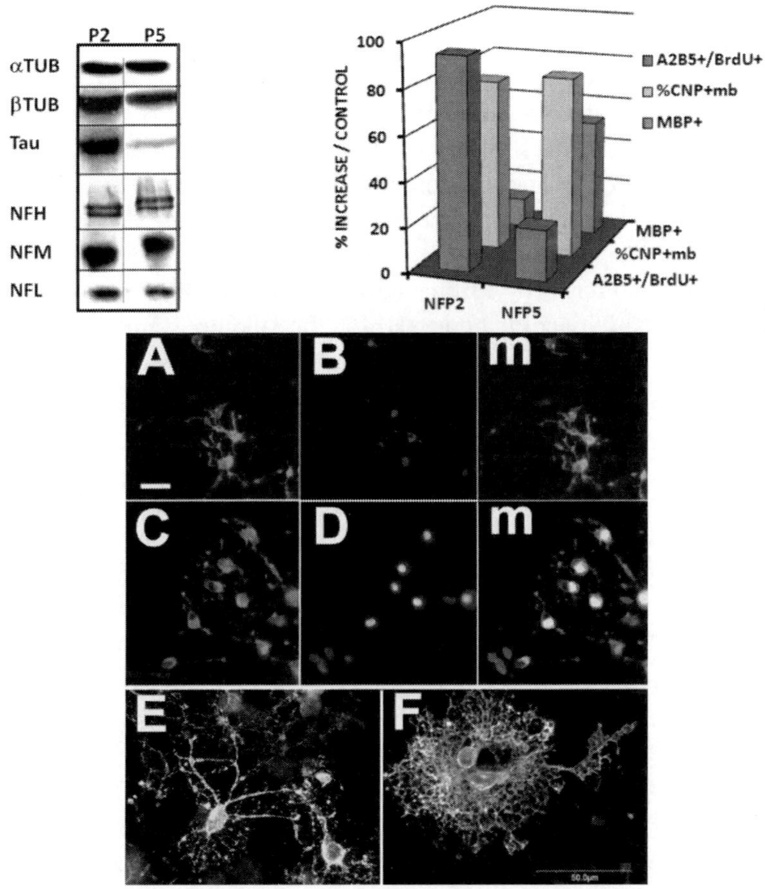

)

Figure 6. Comparison of western blot analysis of the 2nd pellet of NF purification (P2) and of the 5th pellet (P5); some other proteins such as tubulin (TUB) purify with NFP2, whereas NFP5 is highly enriched in the 3 NF subunits (NFL, M, H). Graph depicts differential effects on OL fate of NFP2, which mostly enhanced OLP proliferation (A2B5 +/BrdU + cells, blue bars), and of NFP5 enhancing mainly OL maturation (MBP+ cells, orange bars). Results of immunocytochemistry expressed as percentage of variation compared to untreated controls. Compared to controls (A-B), cultures treated with NFP2 (C-D) contain significantly more proliferating OL progenitors (A2B5 + cells, (A, C)) which have incorporated bromodeoxyuridine (BrdU) in their nuclei, revealed by anti-BrdU mAb (B, D). A2B5 immunostaining revealed with Alexa fluor 488 (A, C), BrdU revealed by Alexa fluor 568 (B, D), and merger of fields (right, m); bar = 20 μm. Neurofilament fractions NFP5 increase OL differentiation and maturation *in vitro*. Compared to controls (E), cultures treated with NF (F) contain significantly more OL with a much differentiated morphology (multiple highly branched processes). MBP immunostaining revealed with Alexa fluor 488; bar = 50 μm.

Strikingly, differentiation also appeared to be stimulated by NFP2 fractions. This was obvious after 3 days: the total number of cells expressing CNP increased, and the relative percentage of cells with a highly differentiated morphology (numerous branched processes and/or membranous extensions (designed as CNP + mb)) also increased by 1.8-fold compared to controls ($p < 0.01$) (Figure 6F). Finally, cell maturation was also enhanced after 3 days by NFP2, since the relative percentage of MBP + cells increased by around 60% ($p < 0.01$) above controls, and MBP + cells had a more complex morphology. The NF fractions obtained by further purification (NFP3-P5) had a different, restricted type of activity compared to NFP2: they did not significantly modify OLP proliferation. Nevertheless, they stimulated OL differentiation and maturation, which increased by more than 80% and 50% respectively ($p < 0.01$).

Other Axon Cytoskeleton Proteins Copurify with NF and Regulate OL Development

Since the effect of NF fractions on OLP proliferation was lost after the second step of NF purification it appeared unlikely that pure NF accounted for it. Therefore, we analyzed which other proteins could associate with NF during the purification procedure. As previously shown (Bocquet et al., 2009), several proteins from the axonal microtubular network, like TUB isoforms, copurify with NF in P2 fractions (Figure 6). In addition, we observed that TUB remained associated with NF through the 4th and 5th purification steps (Figure 6). This was also the case for Tau and microtubule associated proteins (MAPs), which are known to bind to NF (Leterrier et al., 1982, Heiman et al., 1985; Miyata et al., 1986; Hisanaga et al., 1990), as well as spectrin βII (SpbII) (Frappier et al., 1987), and synapsin 2 (SYN2) (Goldenring et al., 1986; Steiner et al., 1987).

To test whether such proteins could account for the proliferation of OL induced by NFP2 fractions, their effects were analyzed separately. Using purified or recombinant proteins we observed that both TUB and MAPs (at 0.1 μg/mL final concentration, corresponding to their estimated concentrations in NFP2) strongly increased OLP proliferation within 24 h (by more than 350% over controls). The other axonal proteins (SYN2, SpbII, and Tau) upregulated also OLP proliferation (A2B5 + /BrdU + cells) within 24 h by two-fold over control (CONT) ($p < 0.01$).

After 3 days all these proteins increased the total number of CNP+ cells with a highly differentiated morphology (CNP + mb). Nevertheless, and contrary to NFP5, the relative percentage of differentiated cells (CNP+) and of mature OL within treated cultures did not significantly differ from CONT. This suggested that OLP had been induced to proliferate during the first 24 h of treatment, and that their differentiation and maturation have been neither delayed nor enhanced then by NF associated proteins.

The specificity of NF fractions and NF associated proteins effects was further evidenced by control experiments with human recombinant glial fibrillary acidic protein (GFAP) (Middeldorp, 2011), purified actin which is known to bind NF (Hao et al., 1997), purified albumin, as well as rat liver, or skin protein extracts. Contrary to NF and NF associated proteins, all these proteins were ineffective on OL cultures. Thus the properties of NF (the intermediate filaments specific to neurons) on OL growth were not shared by other intermediate filament proteins such as GFAP, specific to AS. Similarly the effects of the NF associated proteins TUB, MAPs, Tau, SYN2, SpbII were not recorded with other NF associated proteins, such as actin despite its ability to bind NF (not shown).

The specificity of these effects of NF and axon proteins on cells of the OL lineage was assayed in pure astrocyte (AS) cultures using the same conditions. NF P2 to P5 fractions (50-2000 ng/mL) decreased only slightly (30% below CONT) the proliferation of AS after 24 h, while their morphological differentiation and GFAP expression were not affected (not shown). The other axon cytoskeleton proteins (TUB, MAPs, Tau, SpbII, SYN2) also did not modify AS differentiation as evidenced by morphology and GFAP immunostaining. Nevertheless, they stimulated AS proliferation analyzed by double immunolabeling (GFAP + /BrdU + cells) ranging from 15% (MAPs) to 74% (TUB) over controls (not shown). Thus, this effect was less pronounced than for OLP.

Mechanism of Action and Signaling Pathways of NF and Associated Axon Cytoskeleton Proteins

Subtle morphological changes of the OL cytoskeleton immunolabeled with βTUB (Terada et al., 2005) were observed after 3 days when OL cultures were treated with NF fractions (not shown). Compared to controls there was an increase in the number, length, and complexity of OL processes. Nevertheless, there was no other modification of the OL cytoskeleton. Several putative signaling pathways, known to be involved in the regulation of OL, were explored to characterize the mechanisms of action of NF fractions and their associated proteins. For example, Src family protein expression, to which Fyn kinase belongs, and which is involved in OL process outgrowth (Klein et al., 2002) and in myelination (e.g., Krämer et al., 1999, Sperber et al., 2001; White et al., 2008), was not altered. Similarly, Akt (Flores et al., 2008: Narayanan et al., 2009), pospho-MEK (Boggs et al., 2008), Rho (Liang et al., 2004, Kippert et al., 2007), PTEN and phospho-GSK (Harrington et al., 2010; Azim and Butt, 2011) did not appear to be involved.

Despite the lack of a known receptor other intercellular interactions have been reported in the CNS. For example myelin proteins alter OLP differentiation (Baer et al., 2009), and axolemma-enriched fractions increase OLP proliferation (Becker-Catania et al., 2010). In addition other signaling from neuron to glia has been observed, without evidence of a specific molecular pathway (Trajkovic et al., 2006). Thus, it appears plausible that other types of regulation occur too, as observed between NF and OL. Alternately, structural proteins of the OL, such as PLP and MBP, could act as transducers for external signals (Dyer and Matthieu, 1994; Dyer et al., 1994; Fulton et al., 2010; Macklin et al., 2012). Interestingly novel and unconventional roles for myelin proteins are increasingly identified. These non-structural functions encompass several types, such as calcium channel regulation by proteolipid (PLP), or cytoskeleton binding by MBP and golli proteins for example (review in Fulton et al., 2010). Myelin oligodendrocyte glycoprotein (MOG), one of the main targets of experimental autoimmune encephalitis (EAE), may also activate signaling cascades upon cross-linking with immunoglobulins (Marta et al., 2005). Nevertheless, this mechanism is unlikely to explain the effects of axon proteins on OLP, which do not express myelin proteins. However, given the tight interactions between axons and OL (e.g., Piaton et al., 2009), axon cytoskeleton protein released in the extracellular space could signal to cells of the OL lineage through such types of proteins, and finally trigger proliferation and differentiation resulting in remyelination.

In addition, unconventional interactions between proteins and cells have been demonstrated: intracellular Tau fibrils are released into the media and then taken up by co-cultured cells, resulting in transcellular propagation of Tau aggregation; this mechanism could be involved in neurodegenerative diseases such as Alzheimer's disease (Kfoury et al., 2012). Alternately, some peptides are known as "cell penetrating peptides" (CPP) and lack membrane receptor (Dupont et al., 2007; Proschiantz, 2008). Although partial proteolysis of NF fractions could release biologically active peptides, there is no homology of sequence between NF, or the other axon proteins tested, and these CPP to support this hypothesis. We observed that labeled TUB bound mature OL (Fressinaud et al., 2012), but other labeled cytoskeleton proteins are not yet available, precluding any comparison.

NF and Proteins from the Axon Cytoskeleton Improve Recovery and Prevent OL from LPC Toxicity *In Vitro*

The effects of NF and their associated cytoskeleton proteins on OL growth under basal conditions prompted us to determine whether they could also regulate OL fate under demyelinating conditions, since NF release in the CSF occurs mostly during MS relapses.

Thus, the putative effects of NF and axon proteins to improve OL survival during LPC treatment (24 h) were tested in two conditions: i) to investigate OL recovery: the proteins were added to the CDM after LPC removal, or ii) to search for a protective effect: axon proteins were added at the same time as LPC to the CDM (LPC was removed after 24 h).

Recovery after LPC Is Improved by NF and TUB

NFP2 and TUB Restore OLP Proliferation after LPC

After treatment for 24 h with LPC ($2. 10^{-5}$ M), LPC was removed and cells were either grown in CDM alone, or treated for 1-3 days with NFP2 fractions, or TUB. Phase contrast microscopy observations and immunolabeling after 24 h revealed that NFP2 fractions partially rescued cells from LPC attack. Compared to cultures treated only with LPC the effects of NFP2 were obvious: the number of A2B5 +/BrdU + cells increased by 235%, ($p < 0.01$). Tubulin had similar effects, and the total number of A2B5 +/BrdU + cells increased by 200%, compared to LPC alone ($p < 0.01$). On the contrary, control proteins (actin, skin proteins) were ineffective (not shown, see below).

NFP5 and TUB Restore OL Maturation after LPC Treatment

In these experiments NFP5 fractions, rather than NFP2, were used because they increase maturation under basal conditions (see above). When cells were treated with NFP5 after LPC removal, and contrary to what was observed with LPC alone, the number of CNP+ and MBP+ cells did not differ significantly from untreated controls (no LPC) after 3 days, indicating that NFP5 rescued OL. The effects of NFP5 on cell morphology were evident since a majority of cells extending numerous ramified processes could be observed, contrary to cells treated only with LPC. Compared to LPC alone, NFP5 significantly increased the number of CNP + OL by more than 160% ($p < 0.01$). Maturation was also improved as MBP + OL number increased by 150% versus LPC (not shown). The effects of TUB were weaker than those of NFP5. Differentiation and maturation (CNP + and MBP+ OL number) increased by more than 125% and did not differ significantly from untreated controls when cells were treated with TUB in addition to LPC (not shown). NF and TUB effects on OL differentiation appeared significant and specific since high albumin concentrations (0.5 mg/mL) were present in the CDM and had no effect.

Axon Cytoskeleton Proteins Significantly Prevent OL from LPC Toxicity

Axon Proteins Increase OLP Survival and Their Proliferation When Challenged with LPC, They Partly Preserve OL Differentiation and Maturation

Compared to LPC treatment alone, NFP2 added at the time of LPC increased the number of OLP by 100% after 24 h, and the relative percentage of proliferating cells (ratio of A2B5 + and BrdU + cells to total A2B5+ cells) by 39% ($p < 0.01$) (Figure 7). Similar results were obtained for TUB (Figure 7) which increased total A2B5+ cells (OLP) by 90% compared to LPC alone, and their proliferation by more than 50% ($p < 0.01$). These effects were specific since control proteins (actin and skin proteins) were ineffective (not shown). Combined treatment with NF and TUB did not result in the addition or potentiation of their effects (not shown).

NFP5 treatment added at the time of LPC significantly increased after 3 days the total number of CNP + OL by 65% versus LPC alone (Figure 7), and that of CNP + cells with myelin-like membranes increased by 55%. Maturation (number of MBP + OL) was increased by 150% (Figure 7), ($p < 0.01$). Tubulin also increased differentiation and maturation by more than 140% and 175%, respectively, compared to LPC (Figure 7).

The number of highly differentiated (CNP + mb) OL increased by 135%, and the ratio of mature to differentiated cells (MBP +/CNP +) increased by 55% versus LPC alone. Concomitant addition of NFP5 and TUB to LPC did not increase further differentiation and maturation compared to separate treatments. There was no potentiation of NF and TUB effects.

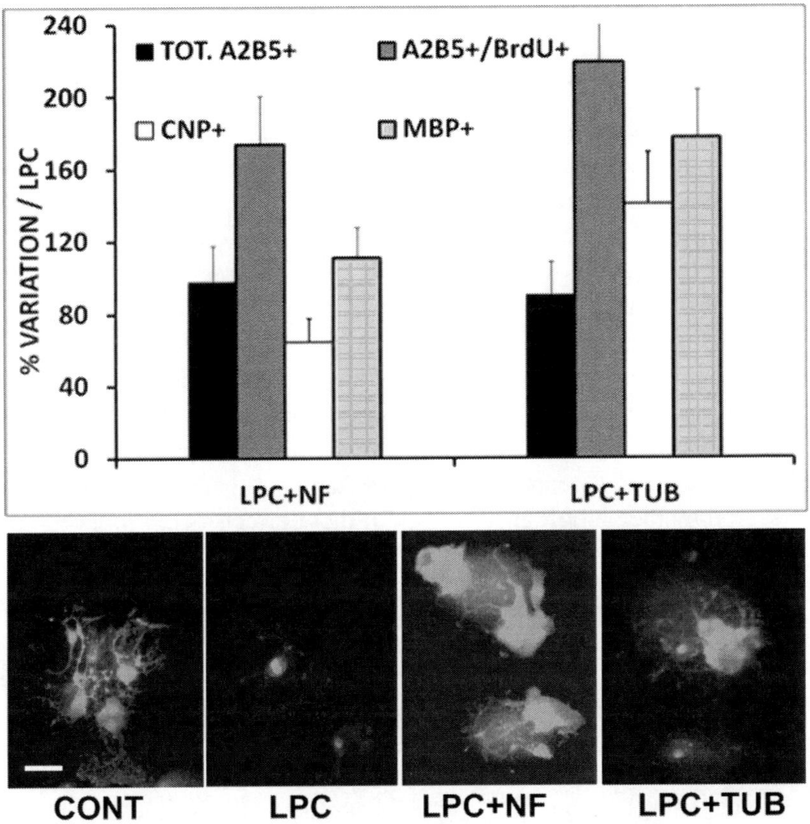

Figure 7. NF and TUB prevent OL from LPC toxicity. Upper panel: results of immunocytochemistry as percentage of variation compared to cultures treated only with LPC (2.10^{-5} M, 24 h). NFP2 was used for analyses of OLP (A2B5+ cells, day 3, black and gray bars), and NFP5 for differentiation and maturation studies (CNP+ and MBP+ cells, day 6, white and light gray bars), TUB was used at day 3 and 6. All the differences are significant ($p < 0.01$). An example of the different conditions (untreated control, LPC alone, LPC and NF or TUB) with CNP immunostaining is presented (lower panel). Bar = 15 µm.

Control proteins (actin, skin proteins) had no detectable effect under these conditions, demonstrating the specificity of NF and TUB effects on OL (not shown). So, as for the rescue experiments, all the parameters analyzed (i.e., proliferation, number of differentiated and of mature cells) were greatly increased by NF and TUB compared to cultures treated with LPC only.

Mechanisms of the Preventive Effects of NF and TUB

Detailed analyses of the cell populations suggest that improved recovery and prevention from LPC toxicity induced by axon cytoskeleton proteins could result mainly from two mechanisms: an increased cell survival, and increased proliferation (NFP2 and TUB), followed rapidly by differentiation. Indeed given the length of the OLP cell cycle (around 25 h (Hyrien et al., 2010)), increased proliferation alone is unlikely to result in such a dramatic increase in OLP number during the time of experiments (24 h). A survival effect of NFP5 appears likely since it did not induce OLP proliferation under standard conditions. The effects of TUB could result from the differentiation of OLP that have been induced to proliferate during the treatment. Under these conditions OLP mature in around 3 days (Fressinaud et al., 1995), and analyses were performed on day 5 (i.e., 3 days after LPC treatment). This supports the hypothesis of the maturation of new progenitors generated during exposition to LPC and TUB. Around from one half up to 100% of OLP and mature OL survive to LPC during prevention and rescue experiments respectively. Thus, this represents an important number of cells of the OL lineage spared by the pathological process if these effects occur *in vivo*.

Synthetic Peptide NFL-TBS.40-63 Corresponding to the Tubulin-binding Site (TBS) Sequence Identified on Light NF Chain Modulates OL Maturation and Remyelination *In Vitro*

To determine more precisely the putative roles of extra-axonal NF we have taken advantage of synthetic peptides corresponding to the sequence that binds tubulin (TBS) on NF light chain (NFL) described in the laboratory (Bocquet et al., 2009; Berges et al., 2012), and we have tested their effects in pure OL cultures. In addition, we have used LPC-induced demyelination (Fressinaud, 2005) to test whether TBS-peptides could improve recovery in this model. Our aim was to explore if this peptide sequence could account for the effects of NF on OL previously reported. We hypothesized also that this peptide might be released or exposed after axon damage during demyelination *in vivo*. Biotinylated peptides (more than 95% purity) were synthesized according to the TBS sequence identified in NFL chain (NFL-TBS.40-63: YSSYSAPVSSSLSVRRSYSSSSGS) and in keratin as control (Ker-TBS.1-24: MSIRVTQKSYKMSTSGPRAFSSRS). Scrambled peptide with the same amino-acids that NFL-TBS.40-63, although in random sequence (NFL-SCR: SLGSPSSSVRASYSSSRSYVYSSS) was also used as a control (lack of TBS site) (Bocquet et al., 2009). Peptides were dissolved in water and used at 10 μM final concentration except where otherwise specified. They were added to rat oligodendrocyte (OL) and astrocyte (AS) cultures, grown in CDM for 1-3 days (basal conditions). In addition, the demyelinating chemical LPC (2. 10^{-5} M, 24 h) was used as described above to induce OL death and to test the effects of TBS-peptides under these demyelinating conditions (Fressinaud and Eyer, 2014).

OL Differentiation and Maturation In Vitro Are Promoted by NFL-TBS.40-63 Peptide

Analyses of OL cultures grown in CDM revealed that the NFL-TBS.40-63 peptide (10 μM) regulated OL development. Its effects were selective, as it increased significantly OL differentiation and maturation, while OLP proliferation was unchanged compared to untreated control cultures (CDM alone). After 24 h of treatment with NFL-TBS.40-63 neither the number of A2B5 + OLP nor that of proliferating (BrdU +) cells was increased compared to untreated controls (Fressinaud and Eyer, 2014) (not shown). On the contrary, three days after treatment with NFL-TBS.40-63, differentiation appeared to be stimulated since the percentage of differentiated (CNP+) cells increased by more than 90% ($p < 0.01$) compared to untreated controls. Moreover, differentiated cells (expressing CNP) and extending membranes or numerous thin branched processes (> 5 ramified processes (CNP + mb)) increased by 120% (not shown). These cells correspond to highly differentiated OL (e.g., Sperber and McMorris, 2001). Finally, cell maturation was also enhanced by the NFL-TBS.40-63 peptide after 3 days, since MBP + cells increased above controls by more than 170% ($p < 0.01$). As for CNP + OL, MBP + cells displayed a more developed shape in peptide-treated cultures than their untreated counterparts. Dose response experiments (1-100 μM) did not reveal significant modifications of the NFL-TBS.40-63 effects, and a maximal response was obtained for 10 μM concentration (not shown).

Effects of Other Peptides and Specificity of NFL-TBS.40-63 Peptide Effects on OL

The scrambled NFL peptide (NFL-SCR2), composed of the same amino-acids as NFL-TBS.40-63 although distributed randomly, did not alter OLP proliferation. It slightly enhanced OL maturation, with an increase in MBP+ cells, which did not reach significance. The KER-TBS.1-24 peptide (corresponding to the TBS of keratin), had similar effects to NFL-TBS.40-63, although to a lower extent. It did not upregulate OLP proliferation.

Nevertheless, it did induce a slight increase in OL with a highly differentiated morphology as well as an increase in the number of mature cells.

To determine whether the effects of the TBS peptides were specific to OL, the same peptides (NFL-TBS.40-63, NFL-SCR2, and KER-TBS.1-24) were assayed in pure AS cultures using the same conditions (1-3 days of treatment in CDM). None of the peptides modified significantly the proliferation nor the differentiation of AS.

Mechanisms of Action and Signaling Pathways

Immunocytological localization of biotinylated peptides revealed by streptavidin, coupled to Alexa-fluor 488 allowed for the assessment of their distribution in the cell body and proximal parts of main processes in CNP+ OL. To ensure proper localization, biotinylated peptides were used at 50 μM final concentration. Quantification confirmed that most of the cells (OLP as well as mature OL) were labeled by NFL-TBS.40-63. This was also confirmed by confocal microscopy (Fressinaud and Eyer, 2014; 2015) (see below and Figure 9). As for NF, several putative signaling pathways were explored to characterize the mechanisms of action of the NFL-TBS.40-63 peptide. The following pathways known to be involved in OL differentiation and myelination were analyzed and did not appear to be involved: i) Src, ii) Akt, iii) Rho, and phospho-MEK, and (iv) PTEN and phospho-GSK.

The NFL-TBS.40-63 Peptide Protects OL from LPC Toxicity In Vitro

Since NF could be released by axon lesion during demyelination in MS, we explored whether NFL-TBS.40-63 peptides could prevent OL injury when cells are exposed at the same time to LPC (e.g., Fressinaud and Eyer, 2013).

As previously described, 2. 10^{-5} M LPC for 24 h (Figure 8) induced the death of half of the cells compared to untreated controls, and there was no spontaneous recovery 2 days later. Also, after LPC treatment, surviving cells displayed an altered morphology with short, truncated ramifications, or lack of processes (Figure 8).

On the contrary, 2 days after LPC removal, in cultures treated simultaneously with LPC and NFL-TBS.40-63 (Figure 8), OL were more numerous and some of the cells had the characteristic multi-process morphology of differentiated OL, as in untreated control cultures. These effects were obvious by simple observation of living cells in culture by phase contrast microscopy, but they were only partial since LPC + NFL-TBS.40-63 treated cells could still be distinguished from untreated controls.

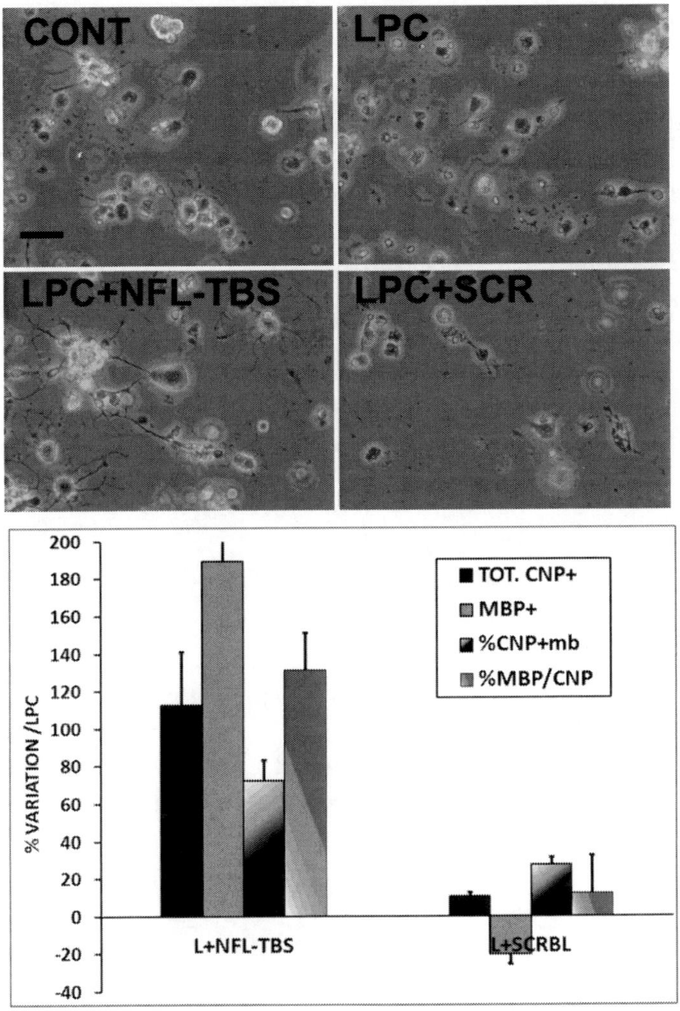

Figure 8. NFL-TBS.40-63 peptides prevent OL from LPC injury *in vitro*, when added at the time of LPC. Phase contrast microscopy of controls, LPC treated cells, OL treated with NFL-TBS.40-63 and LPC, and cells treated with scrambled NFL (inactive peptide (SCR)). NFL-TBS.40-63 allows the survival of more OL with a better preserved morphology, whereas the scrambled peptide is ineffective. Bar = 20 μm. Graph for immunocytochemistry results in percentage of variation compared to LPC alone. Only NFL-TBS.40-63 significantly increases the number and the relative percentage of differentiated (CNP+) and of mature (MBP +). Cells with a highly differentiated morphology (multiple thinly branched processes and/or membranes) correspond to black and gray striped bars (CNP + mb).

This preventive effect of NFL-TBS.40.63 appeared specific since on the contrary, NFL-SCR2 scrambled peptide did not decrease cell death compared to cultures treated with LPC only, and was also unable to improve morphological alterations (Figure 8).

These results were confirmed by immunocytochemistry. Compared to cultures treated with LPC alone (Figure 8 graph), NFL-TBS.40-63 addition resulted in increased number of differentiated and mature cells, evidenced by a 110% increase of the total number of CNP + and CNP + mb OL, while MBP + cells increased by 180% ($p < 0.01$). Since the peptide did not induce OL proliferation this result was suggestive of an enhanced survival, NFL-TBS.40-63 preventing part of the OL from LPC toxicity.

A slight effect was observed with concomitant treatment of cells with LPC and KER-TBS.1-24 (not shown), which increased only the percentage of CNP + mb and of MBP + cells, whereas NFL-SCR2 was inefficient (Figure 8).

Endocytosis of NFL-TBS.40-63 Peptide and Axon Cytoskeleton Proteins by OL

Immunocytochemistry (see above) coupled to confocal microscopy revealed that NFL-TBS.40-63 enters most cells of the OL lineage. The mechanism of entry of these peptides into OL was unknown until recently (Fressinaud and Eyer, 2015). However, in glioblastoma cell lines it has been demonstrated that the NFL-TS.40-63 peptide enters in the cells via endocytosis (Balzeau et al., 2012; Lépinoux-Chambaud and Eyer, 2013).

Recently we demonstrated that NF and TUB, as well as NFL-TBS.40-63 are taken up by endocytosis in OL cultures (Fressinaud and Eyer, 2015). The intracellular localization of the axon proteins and peptides was clearly demonstrated by confocal microscopy (Figure 9). Immunocytochemistry with anti-NFH mAb allowed for the detection of NFP2 in A2B5 + OLP as well as in MBP+ OL.

Similarly, we observed rhodamine (TRITC)-labeled TUB uptake into OL. Endocytosis was characterized in cells in each of the stages of differentiation (progenitors, differentiated, and mature OL). Finally, biotinylated NFL-TBS.40-63 uptake was observed in OLP as well as in differentiated CNP + OL. This endocytic process was confirmed by several markers. So, cholera toxin, a marker of endocytosis, was demonstrated to colocalize in OL with NFL-TBS.40-63.

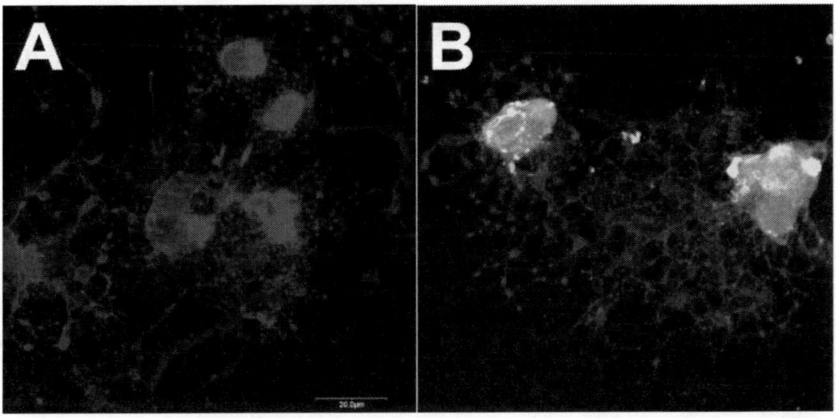

Figure 9. Endocytosis of NFL-TBS.40-63 by OL *in vitro*. (A) Control cultures labeled with anti-CNP Ab (Alexa fluor 568, red), and (B) cultures treated with the peptide: biotinylated NFL-TBS.40-63 peptides (revealed by streptavidine coupled to Alexa-488, green) penetrate into OL labeled with anti-CNP antibody (red),), confocal microscopy, merger of fields, (green and red superposition: yellow). Bar = 20 μm.

This uptake was completely abolished by OL pretreatment with methyl β cyclodextrin which alters lipid rafts and inhibits clathrin and caveolin-dependent endocytosis (Rodal et al., 1999). Furthermore, the uptake of NF and NFL-TBS.40-63 was partly inhibited by dynasore, an inhibitor of dynamin (a GTPase involved in clathrin-dependent endocytosis), indicating clathrin-dependent endocytosis (Henley et al., 1998; Kirchhausen et al., 2008).

Conclusion

In conclusion the NFL-TBS.40-63 peptide specifically increases OL differentiation and maturation *in vitro*, and partly protects them from demyelinating injury. It shares all these properties with the last fraction recovered from NF purification: NFP5, previously reported (Fressinaud et al., 2012; Fressinaud and Eyer, 2013). The homology of sequence with NFL, and their similarity of effects might indicate that NFL-TBS.40-63 accounts for increased differentiation of OL observed with NFP5. On the contrary, TUB, which partly copurifies with NF by binding to TBS, increases OLP proliferation without delaying their differentiation or their maturation *in vitro*. Our results *in vitro* demonstrate that these peptides and proteins exert their proremyelinating activity following endocytosis by cells of the OL lineage.

Importantly, release of such TBS-peptide, or proteolytic fragments of NFL containing this sequence, during axon injury could improve remyelination *in vivo*. We have observed that a single demyelinating event is often followed by remyelination, despite a transient decrease in NF and TUB expression in axons (Jean et al., 2002). We hypothesize that this could correspond to the release by axons of the native, untransformed, subunits of NF containing the NFL-TBS propremyelinating peptide during a first demyelinating event. In that case complete remyelination will occur. In MS lesions, on the contrary, altered NF expression (Trapp et al., 1998; Fressinaud et al., 2005) and abnormal NF proteolysis (Jain et al., 2009) might result in the release of abnormal NF isoforms (e.g., lacking NFL-TBS) with a reduced capacity to stimulate OL. This might impair remyelination after several relapses in MS.

These results point to some OL plasticity, even at the mature stage of differentiation, in response to some growth factors and axon cytoskeleton proteins. These proteins are able to prevent OL from demyelinating insults *in vitro*. This study brings new insights in order to explain the paucity of remyelination in MS, and suggests that the profound alterations of axon cytoskeleton proteins that are observed in MS plaques might, in turn, inhibit remyelination. Better insight into OL/axon crosstalk especially during demyelination/remyelination is needed to avoid prolonged demyelination and major axon damage that appears beyond repair capacities in MS.

Acknowledgment

This work has been supported in part by a PHRC grant from the University Hospital of Angers.

References

Allamargot C., Pouplard-Barthelaix A., Fressinaud C. 2001. A single intracerebral injection of platelet-derived growth factor (PDGF) accelerates the rate of remyelination *in vivo*. *Brain Res*, 918: 28-39.

Azim, K., Butt, A. M. 2011. GSK3β negatively regulates oligodendrocyte differentiation and maturation *in vivo*. *Glia* 59, 540-53.

Baer, A. S., Syed, Y. A., Kang, S. U., Mitteregger, D., Vig, R., Ffrench-Constant, C., Franklin, R. J., Altmann, F., Lubec, G., Kotter, M. R. 2009.

Myelin-mediated inhibition of oligodendrocyte precursor differentiation can be overcome by pharmacological modulation of Fyn-RhoA and protein kinase C signalling. *Brain* 132 (Pt 2), 465-81.

Balzeau J., Peterson A., Eyer J. 2012. The vimentin-tubulin binding site peptide (Vim-TBS.58-81) crosses the plasma membrane and enters the nuclei of human glioma cells. *Int J Pharm*. 423, 77-83.

Becker-Catania, S. G., Nelson, J. K., Olivares, S., Chen, S.-J., De Vries, G. H., 2011. Oligodendrocyte progenitor cells proliferate and survive in an immature state following treatment with an axolemma-enriched fraction. *ASN Neuro* 3(1), art:e00053.doi:10.1042/AN20100035.

Berges R., Balzeau J., Peterson A. C., Eyer J. 2012. A tubulin binding Peptide targets glioma cells disrupting their microtubules, blocking migration, and inducing apoptosis. *Mol Ther*. 20, 1367-1377.

Bitsch, A., Schuchardt, J., Bunkowski, S., Kuhlmann, T., Bruck, W. 2000. Acute axonal injury in multiple sclerosis. Correlation with demyelination and inflammation. *Brain* 123, 1174-1183.

Bocquet, A., Berges, R., Franck, R., Robert, P., Peterson, A.C., Eyer, J. 2009. Neurofilaments bind tubulin and modulate its polymerization. *J. Neurosci.* 29, 11043-11054.

Boggs, J. M., Gao, W., Hirahara, Y. 2008. Signal transduction *J. Neurosci. Res*. 86, 1448-58.

Brück, W., Schmied, M., Suchanek, G., Brück, Y., Breitschopf, H., Poser, S., Piddlesden, S., Lassmann, H. 1994, Oligodendrocytes in the early course of multiple sclerosis, *Ann. Neurol*, 35, 65-73.

Brück, W., Lucchinetti, C., Lassmann, H. 2002, The pathology of primary progressive multiple sclerosis, *Mult. Scler*, 8, 93-97.

Chang, A., Tourtelotte, W. W., Rudick, R., Trapp, B. D. 2002, Premyelinating oligodendrocytes in chronic lesions of multiple sclerosis, *N. Engl. J. Med.* 346, 165-173.

Dashiell, S. M., Tanner, S. L., Pant, H. C., Quarles, R. H. 2002. Myelin-associated glycoprotein modulates expression and phosphorylation of neuronal cytoskeletal elements and their associated kinases. *J. Neurochem.* 81, 1263-1272.

Defaux, A., Zurich, M. G., Honegger, P., Monnet-Tschudi, F., 2010, Inflammatory responses in aggregating rat brain *Brain Res*. 1353, 213-24.

De Luca, G. C., Williams, K., Evangelou, N., Ebers, G. C., Esiri, M. M. 2006, The contribution of demyelination to axonal loss in multiple sclerosis. *Brain* 129, 1507-1516.

Dupont, E., Prochiantz, A., Joliot, A. 2007. Identification of a signal peptide *J. Biol. Chem*. 282, 8994-9000.

Dyer, C. A., Matthieu, J. M. 1994. Antibodies to myelin/oligodendrocyte-specific protein and myelin/oligodendrocyte glycoprotein signal distinct changes in the organization of cultured oligodendroglial membrane sheets. *J. Neurochem*. 62, 777-787.

Dyer, C. A., Philibotte, T. M., Wolf, M. K., Billings-Gagliardi, S. 1994, Myelin basic protein mediates extracellular signals that regulate microtubule stability in oligodendrocyte membrane sheets. *J. Neurosci. Res*. 39, 97-107.

Fasani, F., Bocquet, A., Robert, P., Peterson, A., Eyer, J. 2004. The amount of neurofilaments aggregated in the cell body is controlled by their increased sensitivity to trypsin-like proteases. *J. Cell Sci*. 117, 861-869.

Fisher, I., Konola, J., Cochary, E. 1990. Microtubule associated protein (MAP1B) is present in cultured oligodendrocytes and co-localizes with tubulin. *J. Neurosci. Res*. 27, 112-124.

Flores, A. I., Narayanan, S. P., Morse, E. N., Shick, H. E., Yin, X., Kidd, G., Avila, R. L., Kirschner, D. A., Macklin, W. B. 2008, Constitutively active Akt induces enhanced myelination in the CNS. *J. Neurosci*. 28, 7174-83.

Frappier, T., Regnouf, F., Pradel, L. A., 1987, Binding of brain spectrin to the 70-kDa neurofilament subunit protein, *Eur. J. Biochem*. 169, 651-7.

Fressinaud, C. 2005. Repeated injuries dramatically affect cells of the oligodendrocyte lineage: effects of PDGF and NT-3 *in vitro. Glia* 49, 555-566.

Fressinaud C. 2007. [Oligodendroglial defect and insufficiency of remyelination during MS: Anatomoclinical and experimental comparative study] *Rev Neurol* (Paris) 163, 448-54.

Fressinaud, C., Vallat, J. M. 1994. Basic fibroblast growth factor *J. Neurosci. Res*. 38, 202-213.

Fressinaud, C., Sazdovitch, V. 2007, *Neurofilaments as the central core of axonal damage in MS (relevance for repair)*. In: Multidrug resistance-associated proteins, Aiello, C. V. (Ed), New York, Nova Science Publishers, pp. 137-157.

Fressinaud C, Eyer J. 2013. Axoskeletal proteins *Neurochem Int,* 62, 306-13.

Fressinaud C, Eyer J. 2014. Neurofilament-tubulin binding site peptide NFL-TBS.40-63 increases the differentiation of oligodendrocytes *in vitro* and partly prevents them from lysophosphatidyl choline toxiciy. *J. Neurosci. Res*. 92:243-53.

Fressinaud C, Eyer J. 2015. Neurofilaments and NFL-TBS.40-63 peptide penetrate oligodendrocytes through clathrin-dependent endocytosis to promote their growth and survival *in vitro. Neuroscience* 298:42-51.

Fressinaud, C., Vallat, J. M., Rigaud, M., Cassagne, C., Labourdette, G., Sarliève, L. L. 1990. Investigations of myelination *in vitro*: Polar lipid content and fatty acid composition of myelinating oligodendrocytes in rat oligodendrocyte cultures. *Neurochem. Int.* 16, 27-39.

Fressinaud, C., Laeng, P., Labourdette, G., Durand, J., Vallat, J. M. 1993. The proliferation of mature oligodendrocytes *in vitro* is stimulated by basic fibroblast growth factor and inhibited by oligodendrocyte-type 2 astrocyte precursors. *Dev. Biol.* 158, 317-329.

Fressinaud, C., Vallat, J. M., Labourdette, G., 1995, Basic fibroblast growth factor down-regulates myelin basic protein gene expression and alters myelin compaction of mature oligodendrocytes *in vitro. J. Neurosci. Res.*, 40, 285-93.

Fressinaud, C., Vallat, J. M., Pouplard-Barthelaix, A. 1996, Platelet-derived growth factor partly prevents chemically induced oligodendrocyte death and improves myelin-like membranes repair *in vitro. Glia* 16, 40-50.

Fressinaud, C., Jean, I., Dubas, F. 2005. Modifications des neurofilaments et des microtubules axonaux en fonction du mécanisme lésionnel: étude pathologique et expérimentale. *Rev. Neurol.* (Paris) 161, 55-60.

Fressinaud, C., Berges, R., Eyer, J. 2012. Axon cytoskeleton proteins specifically modulate oligodendrocyte growth and differentiation *in vitro. Neurochem. Int.* 60, 78-90.

Fulton, D., Paez, P.M., Campagnoni, A. T. 2010, The multiple roles of myelin protein genes during the development of the oligodendrocyte. *ASN Neuro* 2(1), art:e00027. doi:10.1042/AN20090051.

Goldenring, J. R., Lasher, R. S., Vallano, M. L., Ueda, T., Naito, S., Sternberger, N. H., Sternberger, L. A., De Lorenzo, R. J. 1986, Association of synapsin I with neuronal cytoskeleton *J. Biol. Chem.* 26118, 8495-504.

Gresle, M. M., Butzkueven, H., Shaw, G. 2011. Neurofilament proteins *Mult. Scler. Int.*, Article ID 315406, doi:10.1155/2011/315406.

Hall, G. F., Lee, V. M., 2005. Neurofilament sidearm proteolysis is a prominent early effect of axotomy in lamprey giant central neurons. *J. Comp. Neurol.* 353, 38-49.

Hao, R., MacDonald, R. G., Ebadi, M., Schmit, J. C., Pfeiffer, R. F., 1997, Stable interaction between G-actin and neurofilament light subunit in dopaminergic neurons. *Neurochem. Int.* 31, 825-834.

Harrington, E. P., Zhao, C., Fancy, S. P. J., Kaing, S., Franklin, R. J. M., Rowitch, D.H. 2010. Oligodendrocyte PTEN is required for myelin and axonal integrity, not remyelination. *Ann. Neurol.* 68, 703-713.

Heimann, R., Shelanski, M. L., Liem, R. K. 1985. Microtubule-associated proteins bind specifically to the 70-kDa neurofilament protein. *J. Biol. Chem.* 260, 12160-12166.

Henley J. R., Krueger E. W., Oswald B. J., McNiven M. A. 1998. Dynamin mediated internalization of caveolae. *J Cell Biol* 141, 85-99.

Hisanaga, S., Hirokawa, N. 1990., Dephosphorylation-induced interactions of neurofilaments with microtubules, *J. Biol. Chem.* 265, 21852-21858.

Hoffman, P. N., Cleveland, D. W. 1988. Neurofilament and tubulin expression recapitulates the developmental program during axonal regeneration: induction of a specific β-tubulin isotype. *Proc. Natl. Acad. Sci. USA* 85, 4530-33.

Huizinga, R., van der Star, B. J., Kipp, M., Jong, R., Gerritsen, W., Clarner, T., Puentes, F., Dijkstra, C. D., van der Valk, P., Amor, S. 2012. Phagocytosis of neuronal debris by microglia *Glia* 603, 422-431.

Hyrien, O., Dietrich, J., Noble, M. 2010. Mathematical and experimental approaches to identify and predict the effects of chemotherapy *Cancer Res.* 70, 10051-10059.

Irvine, K. A., Blakemore, W. F. 2008. Remyelination protects axons from demyelination-associated axon degeneration. *Brain* 131, 1464-1477.

Jean I, Allamargot C, Barthelaix-Pouplard A, Fressinaud C. 2002. Axonal lesions and PDGF-enhanced remyelination in the rat corpus callosum after lysolecithin demyelination. *Neuroreport* 13:627-631.

Jean I., Lavialle C., Barthelaix-Pouplard A., Fressinaud C. 2003. Neurotrophin-3 specifically increases mature oligodendrocyte population and enhances remyelination after chemical demyelination of adult rat CNS. *Brain Res.* 972: 110-118.

Jain, M.R., Bian, S., Liu, T., Hu, J., Elkabes, S., Li, H. 2009. Altered proteolytic events in experimental autoimmune encephalomyelitis discovered by iTRAQ shotgun proteomics analysis of spinal cord. *Proteome Sci* 7, 25.doi: 10.1186/1477-5956-7-25.

Kfoury, N., Holmes, B. B., Jiang, H., Holtzman, D. M., Diamond, M. I., 2012. Trans-cellular propagation of Tau aggregation by fibrillar species, *J. Biol. Chem.* 287, 19440-19451.

Kippert, A., Trajkovic, K., Rajendran, L., Ries, J., Simons, M. 2007. Rho regulates membrane transport *J. Neurosci.* 27, 3560-70.

Kirchhausen T., Macia E., Pelish H. E. 2008, Use of dynasore, the small molecule inhibitor of dynamin, in the regulation of endocytosis, *Methods Enzymol* 438, 77-93.

Klein, C., Krämer, E.-M., Cardine, A.-M., Schraven, B., Brandt, R., Trotter, J. 2002, Process outgrowth of oligodendrocytes is promoted by interaction of Fyn kinase with the cytoskeletal protein Tau. *J. Neurosci.* 22, 698-707.

Krämer, E.-M., Klein, C., Koch, T., Boytinck, M., Trotter, J. 1999. Compartmentation of Fyn kinase with glycosylphosphatidylinositol-anchored molecules in oligodendrocytes facilitates kinase activation during myelination. *J. Biol. Chem.* 274, 29042-29049.

Kuhle, J., Leppert, D., Petzold, A., Regeniter, A., Schindler, C., Mehling, M., Anthony, D. C., Kappos, L., Lindberg, R. L. 2011. Neurofilament heavy chain in CSF correlates with relapses and disability in multiple sclerosis. *Neurology* 76, 1206-13.

Lepinoux-Chambaud C., Eyer J. 2013. The NFL-TBS.40-63 anti-glioblastoma peptide enters selectively in glioma cells by endocytosis. *Int J Pharm* 454, 738-47.

Leterrier, J. F, Liem, R. K., Shelanski, M. L. 1982. Interactions between neurofilaments and microtubule-associated proteins: a possible mechanism for intraorganellar bridging. *J. Cell Biol.* 95, 982-986.

Liang, X., Draghi, N. A., Resh, M. D. 2004, Signaling from integrins to Fyn to Rho family GTPases regulates morphologic differentiation of oligodendrocytes. *J. Neurosci.* 24, 7140-7149.

Lycke, J. N., Karlsson, J. E., Andersen, O., Rosengren, L. E. 1998, Neurofilament protein in cerebrospinal fluid: a potential marker of activity in multiple sclerosis. *J. Neurol. Neurosurg. Psychiatry* 64, 402-404.

Macklin, W. B., Harlow, D. E., Vesely, E. M., Komuro, H. 2012, Endogenous and environmental regulators of oligodendrocyte progenitor cell migration. Abstr C10-04, *Trans. Am. Soc. Neurochem.* pp. 39-40.

Marta, C. B., Montano, M. B., Taylor, C. M., Taylor, A. L., Bansal, R., Pfeiffer, S. E. 2005, Signaling cascades *J. Biol. Chem.*, 280, 8985-93.

Mason J. L., Toews A., Hostettler J. D., Morell P., Suzuki K., Goldman J. E., Matsushima GK. 2004. Oligodendrocytes *Am J Pathol.*164, 1673-82.

Mews, I., Bergmann, M., Bunkowski, S., Gulotta, F., Brück, W. 1998. Oligodendrocyte and axon pathology in clinically silent multiple sclerosis lesions. *Mult. Scler.* 4, 55-62.

Middeldorp, J., Hol, E. M. 2011. GFAP in health *Prog. Neurobiol,* 93, 421-443.

Miyata, Y., Hoshi, M., Nishida, E., Minami, Y., Sakai, H. 1986. Binding of microtubule-associated protein 2 and tau to the intermediate filament reassembled from neurofilament 70-kDa subunit protein. Its regulation by calmodulin, *J. Biol. Chem.* 261, 13026-13030.

Narayanan, S. P., Flores, A. I., Wang, F., Macklin, W. B. 2009, Akt signals *J. Neurosci.* 29, 6860-70.

Ozawa, K., Suchanek, G., Breitschopf, H., Brück, W., Budka, H., Jellinger, K., Lassmann, H. 1994. Patterns of oligodendroglia pathology in multiple sclerosis. *Brain* 117, 1311-1322.

Penderis J, Shields S. A., Franklin R. J., 2003. Impaired remyelination *Brain;* 126 (Pt 6), 1382-91.

Piaton, G., Williams, A., Seilhean, D., Lubetzki, C. 2009, Remyelination in multiple sclerosis. *Progress Brain Res.* 175, 453-64.

Prochiantz, A. 2008. Protein and peptide *Adv. Drug Deliv. Rev.* 60, 448-51.

Rodal S. K., Skretting G., Garred O., Vilhardt F., van Deurs B., Sandvig K. 1999. Extraction of cholesterol with methyl-beta-cyclodextrin perturbs formation of clathrin-coated endocytic vesicles. *Mol Biol Cell* 104, 961-974.

Rodriguez, M., Scheithauer, B. W., Forbes, G., Kelly, P. 1993. Oligodendrocyte injury is an early event in lesions of multiple sclerosis. *Mayo Clin. Proc.* 68, 627-636.

Schirmer, L., Antel, J. P., Brück, W., Stadelmann, C. 2011. Axonal loss and neurofilament phosphorylation *Brain Pathol.* 21, 428-440.

Sperber, R. B., Boyle-Walsh, E., Engleka, M. J., Gadue, P., Peterson, A. C., Stein, P. L., Scherer, S. S., McMorris, F. A. 2001. A unique role for Fyn in CNS myelination. *J. Neurosci.* 21, 2039-2047.

Steiner, J. P., Ling, E., Bennett, V. 1987. Nearest neighbor analysis for brain synapsin I. Evidence from *in vitro* reassociation assays for association with membrane protein(s) and the Mr = 68,000 neurofilament subunit. *J. Biol. Chem.* 262, 905-914.

Terada, N., Kidd, G. J., Kinter, M., Bjartmar, C., Moran-Jones, K., Trapp, B. D., 2005. βIV Tubulin is selectively expressed by oligodendrocytes in the central nervous system. *Glia* 50, 212-222.

Teunissen, C. E., Dijkstra, C., Polman, C., 2005. Biological markers in CSF and blood for axonal degeneration in multiple sclerosis. *Lancet Neurol.* 4, 32-41.

Trajkovic, K., Dhaunchak, A. S., Goncalves, J. T., Wenzel, D., Schneider, A., Bunt, G., Nave, K. A., Simons, M. 2006. Neuron to glia *J. Cell Biol.* 172, 937-48.

Trapp, B. D., Peterson, J., Ransohof, R. M., Rudick, R., Mörk, S., Bö, L. 1998. Axonal transection in the lesions of multiple sclerosis, *N. Engl. J. Med.* 338, 278-285.

Waxman S. G., Kocsis J. D., Nitta K. C. 1979. Lysophosphatidyl choline *J Neurol Sci.* 44, 45-53.

White, R., Gonsior, C., Krämer-Albers, E. M., Stöhr, N., Hüttelmaier, S., Trotter, J. 2008. Activation of oligodendroglial Fyn kinase enhances translation of mRNAs transported in hnRNP A2-dependent RNA granules. *J. Cell Biol.* 181, 579-586.

Wolswijk G. 2000. Oligodendrocyte survival, loss and birth in lesions of chronic-stage multiple sclerosis. *Brain.* 123 (Pt 1), 105-15.

In: Oligodendrocytes
Editor: Dana Swanson

ISBN: 978-1-63483-330-1

Chapter 5

Role of S100B on Oligodendrocyte Physiology and Pathology

Andreia Barateiro[1], Gisela Santos[1], Vera Afonso[1], Dora Brites[1,2] and Adelaide Fernandes[1,2,*]

[1]Research Institute for Medicines (iMed.ULisboa), Faculty of Pharmacy, Universidade de Lisboa, Lisbon, Portugal

[2]Department of Biochemistry and Human Biology, Faculty of Pharmacy, Universidade de Lisboa, Lisbon, Portugal

Abstract

S100B, a Ca^{2+}-binding protein, is expressed mainly by astrocytes and maturing oligodendrocytes within the central nervous system (CNS). Intracellular S100B stimulates cell proliferation and migration, while at the extracellular level engages a few receptors with different outcomes depending on concentration, cell type and microenvironment. In the CNS, S100B promotes neuroprotection at low levels but if highly expressed may increase glial reactivity and induce brain damage. Although the

[*] Corresponding author: Adelaide Fernandes, Research Institute for Medicines (iMed.ULisboa), Faculty of Pharmacy, Universidade de Lisboa, Av. Professor Gama Pinto, 1649-003 Lisbon, Portugal, Phone: +351217946450; Fax: +351217946491, E-mail: amaf@ff.ulisboa.pt.

effects of S100B on astrocytes, microglia and immune cells have been highly explored, only a few more recent reports implicate S100B in oligodendrocyte physiology and pathology. Here we describe S100 proteins, the intracellular and extracellular effect of S100B on CNS cells, namely in oligodendrogenesis, and its involvement in myelin-related disorders. Furthermore, we highlight the association of increased S100B concentration in the serum and cerebrospinal fluid of patients suffering from myelin-related disorders and shed some light on the mechanisms of S100B-induced myelin injury. Finally, we discuss the potential use of anti-S100B therapies to treat these disorders in order to reduce damage and improve recovery, as well as the quality of life of these patients.

Keywords: myelin, oligodendrocyte, S100B

1. Introduction

S100 proteins were first described in 1965 by Moore *et al.,* which isolated subcellular fraction from bovine brain. This fraction was named S100 since proteins are 100% soluble in ammonium sulphate at neutral pH [1]. Further investigations demonstrated that this fraction contained two polypeptides, S100α (S100A1) and S100β (S100B). S100 proteins, known Ca^{2+}-binding molecules, have been implicated in several cellular physiological function and lately in pathophysiological mechanisms [2].

S100B is now emerging as a biomarker of brain damage, usually associated to astrogliosis [3]. Although astrocytes are the main producers of S100B within the central nervous system (CNS) [4], intracellular oligodendrocyte expression is necessary for proper oligodendrocyte differentiation and maturation [5], while damaged oligodendrocytes release increased levels of S100B [6].

Oligodendrocytes are responsible for CNS myelination and proper oligodendrogenesis is required for accurate formation of brain and spinal cord white matter. Most attractively, cumulative data show increased levels of S100B in serum and cerebrospinal fluid (CSF) of patients suffering from myelin-related disorders [7], suggesting that this molecule play a crucial role in oligodendrocyte physiology and pathology. Here, we introduce S100 proteins, describe the intracellular and extracellular action of S100B on CNS cells, highlighting S100B presence in fluid specimens of patients suffering from myelin-related disorders and shedding some light on potential mechanisms of S100B-induced myelin injury. We also discuss how a S100B-target therapeutic strategy may reduce the damage or improve recovery of myelin lesions.

2. S100 Proteins

S100 proteins belong to a multigenic family of small proteins (approximately 10 kDa) characterized by the presence of two Ca^{2+}-binding sites of the EF-hand type (i.e., helix-loop-helix) interconnected by an intermediate region often referred to as the hinge region. In S100 proteins, while the Ca^{2+}-binding loop located in the N-terminal half is unconventional, in that it is longer rearranged, the other one, located in the C-terminal half is canonical [8]. Consequently, the two Ca^{2+}-binding sites have different affinities to Ca^{2+}, being the C-terminal site the one with higher affinity when compared with the N-terminal site that has a much lower Ca^{2+} affinity (approximately 100-times lower) [9]. S100 C-terminal affinity to Ca^{2+} is normally formed by the 12 residues, characterized by a dissociation constant of about 10-50 μM. On the other hand, Ca^{2+} binds to N-terminal region of S100 proteins with about 14 residues mainly through a chain of carbonyl groups, presenting a dissociation constant of about 200-500 μM. This difference in dissociation constants between C- and N-terminal explains the different Ca^{2+} affinities of S100 proteins. Furthermore, some S100 proteins are also able to bind Zn^{2+}, with a relatively high affinity, and Cu^{2+} [10].

Although first described in the brain [1], S100 proteins are not restricted to the nervous tissue. At present, at least 25 members of this family have been identified, which are exclusively expressed in vertebrates and exhibit somewhat cell-specific distribution that points to specialized roles evolved late in evolution [11]. S100 members differ from one another mostly for the C-terminal extension, length and sequence of the hinge region, which may underlie the specificity of the biological activity of individual proteins. Despite of their larger size, three proteins - filaggrin, trichohyalin and repetin – have been included in S100 family, as they exhibit an S100-like motif along their primary sequence [12, 13]. Of the 25 human S100 proteins, 21 family members (S100A1 to S100A18, filaggrin, trichohyalin and repetin) have genes clustered at chromosome locus 1q21, known as the epidermal differentiation complex [8]. Other gene locations include chromosome 7q22-q3 (S100A11P), 21q22 (S100B), Xp22 (S100G), 4p16 (S100P) and 5q14 (S100Z) [8].

A unique feature of S100 family members is their ability to form homodimers and heterodimers with another S100 member. Within cells, most of S100 proteins exist as homodimers in which the two monomers are related by a two-fold axis of rotation and are held together by non-covalent bonds. However, some S100 proteins form heterodimers with other S100 members, as in specific cases like S100A1/S100B, S100A8/S100A9, S100B/S100A6, S100A1/S100A4 and S100B/S100A11 dimers [14]. Moreover, the ability of these proteins to form non-covalent homodimers and heterodimers makes them dynamic proteins that are able of undergoing through different conformational changes, depending on the type of monomers and on the cell type where they are located. In fact, dimerization of S100 proteins seems important for their biological activities since one S100 monomer is not enough for efficient binding to a target protein. In terms of structure, Ca^{2+} binding induces a remarkable change of the interhelical angle between helix III and IV [15], which leads to swing out of hinge region. In addition, a cleft forms in each monomer that is defined by residues in the hinge region, helices III and IV and the C-terminal extension. These residues have an important role for Ca^{2+}-dependent recognition of S100 target proteins. All these exclusive features that distinguish S100 super family, allow each protein to be differentially distributed and to play a wide variety of functions.

S100 proteins show normally a cell and tissue specific expression pattern, which points toward a high specification. A good example is S100B, which in CNS is predominantly expressed in astrocytes, and to a lesser extent, in neurons, microglia, and oligodendrocytes [16, 17]. On the other hand, S100A1 protein has a broader expression and can be found in cardiomyocytes, slow-twitch skeletal muscle cells, salivary epithelial cells, renal cells and hippocampal neurons. The other small proteins of this family have a more restricted tissue and/or cellular expression [18].

As referred before, the members of S100 family are primarily Ca^{2+} sensor proteins, which once activated by the second messenger Ca^{2+}, interact with a wide range of target proteins involved mainly in cytoskeleton assembly and cell proliferation, thereby regulating their activities. Moreover, S100 proteins can also modulate enzyme activity, Ca^{2+} homeostasis, cell growth and mobility, cell cycle regulation, cell differentiation and cell survival [19]. The exceptions are S100A10 that present regulatory functions independently of intracellular Ca^{2+} concentrations, since it lacks a functional EF-hand Ca^{2+}-binding domain [20], and S100G, which is a Ca^{2+}-modulator protein involved in cytosolic Ca^{2+} buffering [21]. At the extracellular level, S100 proteins interact with cell surface receptors, including receptor for advance glycation end products (RAGE) and toll-like receptors (TLR), and are involved in signal transduction [19].

S100 proteins do not have intrinsic catalytic activity. These proteins undergo conformational changes, as described before, and modulate biological activity by interacting with specific targets via Ca^{2+} binding [22]. In resting cells, when intracellular Ca^{2+} concentration is low, S100 proteins present a hydrophilic conformation [23]. However, increased Ca^{2+} levels, observed during cellular activation due to Ca^{2+} influx through ion channels and/or endoplasmic or sarcoplasmic reticulum release, lead to conformational changes in S100 α-helices, which in turn trigger the exposure of hydrophobic sites enabling the interaction with potential targets [24]. Till know, several targets for S100 proteins have been described, such as enzymes, cytoskeleton components, transcription factors, unsaturated fatty acids, channels, receptors, scaffolding proteins, signaling molecules and TLR ligands [19].

S100 secretion can also occur by stimulation of specific cell activators. However, the mechanism of S100 release remains unclear since these proteins are not secreted via the classical Golgi pathway. Possible mechanisms of nonclassical secretion include translocation across the plasma membrane once these proteins have diverse affinities to lipid structures and vesicular release in neutrophil extracellular traps [25, 26]. Since secreted S100 proteins have all their Ca^{2+}-binding domains occupied, all their functions will depend on other properties, such as their ability to form oligomers, or their ability to bind to transition metals like Zn^{2+}, Cu^{2+} or Mn^{2+}, which may mediate they activity, instead of Ca^{2+} binding [27].

Finally, extracellular action of S100 proteins can similarly be mediated by the interaction with membrane localized proteins, such as ion channels and receptors. Although several receptors have been implicated, many effects are mediated by RAGE. This receptor binds and signals a number of S100 proteins, including S100A1, S100A2, S100A5, S100A6, S100A7, S100A8/A9, S100A11, S100A12, S100A13, S100B, and S100P in a large number of cell types [28, 29]. In this context, structural studies of some S100 proteins demonstrated the existence of at least three recognition sites within two distinct surfaces, which may accommodate multiple binding partners that result in complex interactions, or binding to specific ligands on different target cells [30]. This is supported by studies reporting that some S100 functions that reside within the divergent hinge domains between the Ca^{2+}-binding regions are mimicked by relevant peptides whereas others require homo- or hetero-S100 complexes [31]. Both the chromosomal and cellular locations as well as the reported activities that S100 proteins modulate are summarized in Table 1.

Table 1. S100 proteins and their functions

Name	Proposed Functions
S100A1	Cell growth, energy metabolism and contraction [77, 230]
S100A2	Cell cycle progression and differentiation, organization of actin cytoskeleton and inhibition of tumor cell motility [231]
S100A3	Epithelial cell differentiation [232]
S100A4	Cell survival and motility, cell migration and invasion dynamics of myosin filaments, neurite extension and angiogenesis [233]
S100A5	Unknown
S100A6	Cell proliferation, cytoskeletal dynamics and tumorigenesis [103]
S100A7	Antimicrobial responses and innate immunity [234]
S100A8/S100A9	Myeloid cell maturation, migration, chemotaxis, degranulation, phagocytosis and respiratory burst of activated granulocytes and monocytes, inflammation and wound repair [235, 236]
S100A10	Intracellular trafficking of target proteins, inflammation, angiogenesis, blood coagulation, macrophage recruitment and migration of tumour-promoting macrophages and [237, 238]
S100A11	Cell growth, intracellular trafficking of target proteins and cytoskeleton-mediated cellular events [239]
S100A12	Interactions between cytoskeletal elements and membranes, neurite extension, epithelial cell growth arrest and inflammatory processes and immune response [240, 241]
S100A13	Intracellular translocation, inflammatory processes and angiogenesis [242, 243]
S100A14	Dual role in tumor cells [244]
S100A16	Adipogenesis [245]
S100B	Neurite extension, cell death, energy metabolism, cell cycle [32]
S100G	Cytosolic Ca^{2+} levels and transport of proteins through membranes [246]
S100P	Cell proliferation and transendothelial migration of tumor cells, tumor growth, drug resistance and metastasis [247]
S100Z	Unknown
Filaggrin, Repetin, Trychohyalin	Lateral interaction of keratin intermediate filaments [12, 13, 248]

In sum, taking into account the wide distribution of S100 proteins, their great variability of functions and important role in the regulation of several physiological events, deregulations in protein concentrations are usually associated to pathological conditions, turning them into promising biomarkers for diagnosis and prognosis of diverse diseases.

3. S100B

As mentioned, S100B was the first member to be identified [1]. It is a Ca^{2+}-binding protein of 92 residues and is the only member of S100 family found on chromosome 21, on the locus 21q22 [32]. S100B consists primarily of S100 BB homodimers, but it can also form heterodimers of β subunits with S100A1 [33], originating the heterocomplex S100B/S100A1 with physiological functions distinct from the respective homodimers [34]. S100B is able to bind two Ca^{2+} ions per monomer (10.5 kDa), but the affinities are altered in the presence of a target protein [35]. Moreover, it was described that S100B has also a high affinity to Zn^{2+} [36], which changes the affinity of the protein to Ca^{2+}, as well as the interaction with usual target proteins. S100B three-dimensional structures have been reported for the Ca^{2+} free [37] and Ca^{2+} bound protein, for both Ca^{2+} and Zn^{2+} bound protein [38], as well as for complexes with several peptides from target proteins [39, 40]. All these structures display a homodimeric protein (21 kDa) and the affinity is so high that monomers are absent under relevant biological situations [41]. However, it was recently described that the conversion of S100B dimer into tetramer and higher oligomers requires a low molecular weight trigger, such as p53, being the tetramers the most kinetically stable form [42]. However, the causes of tetramer formation *in vivo* are unclear, if there are different low molecular weight triggers or whether interaction with targets like its receptor RAGE is necessary.

S100B is the most common S100 protein found in the brain, and makes up approximately 0.5% of all cerebral proteins. Within the CNS and under physiological states, S100B is mainly expressed by astrocytes, while low levels are found in some neuronal populations, microglia, and oligodendrocytes [16, 17]. Astrocytes present an average concentration of about 10 μM of the S100B protein [4], which is released constitutively [43], or increasingly secreted upon stimulation by several agents [44, 45]. The S100B expression varies along development, being first detected in the brain tissue at embryonic day 14. High levels are found at birth and a slight decrease is observed in the days thereafter, although it was shown to proportionally increase with growth and development of CNS until adulthood, when S100B levels stabilize. In addition to CNS cells, S100B is expressed at a variable abundance in a restricted number of cell types, such as kidney epithelial cells, pituicytes, ependymocytes, chondrocytes, adipocytes, melanocytes, Langerhans cells, dendritic cells, certain lymphocyte subpopulations, skeletal myofibres, myoblasts and muscle satellite cells [19].

S100B physiological concentration is necessary for development, plasticity, and damage repair [46]. However, S100B levels are highly conditioned by external factors stimulation and are positively associated with age, since increased S100B concentrations have been detected in various neurodegenerative and neuroinflammatory diseases. Indeed, cellular and tissue distribution of S100B is altered in several neuropathological conditions, including those induced by environmental stressors, infection, trauma and stroke [4]. In contrast, decreased S100B expression may be triggered by external factors that, at least in astrocytes, may involve high levels of glucose, glutamate and interferon (IFN)-γ [44, 47].

Both high levels of S100B and its diffuse cytoplasmic localization allowed the description of the interaction of this protein with several targets such as enzymes and respective substrates, transcription factors and cytoskeleton components. This ability translates into an equally wide variety of Ca^{2+}-dependent regulation of cellular functions, like cell proliferation and differentiation, cell morphology, protein phosphorylation, enzymatic activity, intracellular Ca^{2+} homeostasis, transcription and protection against oxidative damage [32]. Besides being implicated in the regulation of intracellular activities, S100B can also exhibit cytokine-like activity being secreted into extracellular fluids and found in serum, thereby affecting cellular activities in a paracrine, autocrine and endocrine manner [48, 49]. Initially, S100B detected in the extra cytoplasmic space was thought to be released by injured cells; however, it is now known that certain cell types actively secrete this protein, although through a mechanism that is not fully understood [50]. Indeed, S100B protein may cross the blood-brain barrier and can be found in various body fluids like CSF, peripheral blood, umbilical cord blood, amniotic fluid, urine and saliva. Some of these fluids are of easy access, which facilitates the use of S100B as a pathological biomarker. At low physiological levels, S100B play a trophic and protective role on neurons, protecting neurons from stress-induced apoptosis and regulating neurite outgrowth, dopaminergic and glutamatergic synaptic function, in addition to synaptogenesis and long-term plasticity [51-53]. In contrast, high levels of S100B represent a risk of toxicity to these cells, promoting the expression of proinflammatory cytokines and inflammatory stress-related enzymes, such as inducible nitric oxide synthase (iNOS) [54] that induces neuronal dysfunction and apoptosis of neurons and astrocytes [55]. In fact, both intracellular and extracellular concentrations of this protein have been used as markers of glia damage, resulting from compromised/dying astroglial or oligodendroglial cells with ability to activate the response of immune cells, like microglia [54].

3.1. S100B Intracellular Roles

Within CNS, S100B is extensively expressed by astrocytes and some oligodendrocytes of hippocampus and brain cortex, although it can also be present in certain neuronal subpopulations [56, 57]. Moreover, Ca^{2+} signaling is the major cellular response of glial cells upon neuronal activity, rendering intracellular S100B as a putative link between Ca^{2+} signaling and cellular responses [58, 59].

The presence of increased levels of S100B in certain tumour cells led to consider that it should be implicated in cell proliferation and survival events [60]. In fact, it was shown that S100B influences the cell division pathway by binding and activating, in a Ca^{2+}-dependent manner, a serine/threonine protein kinase, the nuclear Dbf2-related kinase, which is implicated in the regulation of cell division and morphology [61]. In addition, S100B inhibits tumour suppressor p53 phosphorylation and consequently its activation, in a Ca^{2+}-dependent manner [62]. Also, intracellular S100B down-regulates p53 expression and vice-versa, which increase cell proliferation [63].

S100B has been shown to impair neuronal and astroglial differentiation through activation of phosphoinositide-3-kinase (PI3K) and respective downstream signaling pathways [64, 65]. However, after differentiation, increased levels of S100B expression do not reverse the phenotype [65]. These facts are supported by the observation of fluctuations in S100B levels among early and late developmental stages suggesting that protein increased expression occurs during the final stages of astrocytic differentiation [66]. Conversely, S100B negative effects on cell differentiation can also occur after binding, and consequently inhibit EAG1 K^+ channels in a Ca^{2+}-dependent manner [67].

Although the majority of the S100B protein is located within the cytoplasm as a soluble form, about 7% is bound to intracellular membranes, the centrosomes, microtubules and type III intermediate filaments [19]. So, S100B seems to play an important role in the assembly of key components of cell cytoarchitecture. Indeed, several studies have already demonstrated that S100B regulates the assembly and disassembly of microtubules in a Ca^{2+}- and pH-dependent manner [68, 69]. In addition, disassembly of microtubules results in enhanced S100B release [70]. To note that this protein is also an inhibitor of the assembly of type III intermediate filaments, such as glial fibrillary acidic protein (GFAP) and desmin [71, 72]. It is suggested that S100B is involved in actomyosin stabilization since this protein interacts with caldesmon inhibiting its phosphorylation by cdc2 kinase and extracellular signal-regulated kinase 1 and 2 (ERK1/2) mitogen-activated protein kinase (MAPK) [73] and consequently the actomyosin ATPase activity [74]. Additionally, S100B can modulate cell cytoarchitecture by interaction with IQGAP1, a small GTPase Cdc42 and Rac1 effector [75, 76], and acting upstream of the PI3K/Akt/RhoA/ROCK axis, favouring stress fibre formation [76].

Another important function of intracellular S100B is the regulation of several enzyme activities. Upregulation of S100B may increase the intracellular energy supply by activating fructose-1,6-bisphosphate aldolase (glycolysis) and phosphoglucomutase (glycogenolysis) [77, 78]. S100B is also considered to play a role in energy metabolism and in dark adaptation by stimulation of membrane bound guanylate-cyclase in photoreceptors [79]. Moreover, S100B is a well-known inhibitor of protein phosphorylation, as it interacts with kinases, blocking their access to substrates [80]. This type of interaction is characteristic of many S100B target proteins, such as neuromodulin growth associated protein 43 (GAP-43), GFAP, annexin-II and tau proteins [78]. Although the mechanisms remain still unknown, more recent studies suggest that S100B interacts with dopamine D_2 receptor leading to ERK1/2 activation and inhibition of adenylyl cyclase activity [81]. However, it is known that D_2 activation in astrocytes result in neurotrophic factors release [82, 83].

3.2. S100B Extracellular Roles

Although expressed by astrocytes in a constitutive manner [84], S100B secretion is regulated by several external factors and conditions. It is known that tumour necrosis factor (TNF)-α, interleukin (IL)-1β, serotonin, lysophosphatidic acid, as well as high levels of cytosolic Ca^{2+}, low levels of glutamate, metabolic stress and serum deprivation enhance S100B release [44, 70, 85]. On the other hand, high levels of glutamate and glucose, inhibition of Src kinase activity, Ca^{2+} channel blockade and gap junction inhibition reduce S100B secretion [86-89].

Extracellular S100B effects are mediated in the brain mostly by binding to its receptor RAGE [29]. RAGE is a member of the immunoglobulin-like cell surface receptor super family, which is primarily involved in inflammation, nephropathy, neurodegeneration and cancer. It is composed by an extracellular moiety, with one N-terminal V-type and two C-type Ig domains, a single transmembrane spanning helix and a short cytosolic domain, which is necessary for signal transduction [90]. RAGE is expressed in several cell types, including neurons, and its ligation by S100B on these cells has been shown to be somehow responsible for protein dual roles. However, RAGE may not be the sole S100B receptor. In fact, recent studies performed in myoblast cells identified fibroblast growth factor receptor 1 as a receptor for mediating S100B mitogenic effects through interaction with fibroblast growth factor 2 [91, 92].

Under physiological conditions, nanomolar levels of S100B are present in the brain extracellular space and play a neuroprotective role (Figure 1). At this concentration S100B is known to exert trophic effects on neurons, by stimulation of neurite extension and regeneration via activation of cdc42-Rac1, by induction of neurogenesis and by increasing neuron survival during development and after injury [93]. S100B is able to protect neuronal cells towards neurotoxic stimuli through upregulation of the anti-apoptotic factor Bcl-2 mediated by activation of ERK1/2 and nuclear factor kappaB (NF-κB) signaling [94]. In addition, S100B can protect neuron injury indirectly since it stimulates neurotoxic glutamate uptake and reduces neurotoxin-mediated activation of microglia and astrocytes [95, 96]. Beside neurons, extracellular S100B acts on astrocytes in an autocrine way. At nanomolar levels S100B stimulates proliferation by phosphorylation of ERK1/2, iNOS activity and mRNA levels due to activation of NF-kB [97-99]. In addition, low S100B concentrations attenuate activation of microglia after stimulation with the neurotoxicant trimethyltin chloride via the signal transducer and activator of transcription 3 (STAT3) pathway [100]. Under stressful conditions S100B tends to be secreted in higher amounts reaching concentrations in the order of micromolar levels, becoming toxic for neurons and glial cells (Figure 1). In this context, high S100B values were shown to kill neurons through excessive production of reactive oxygen species (ROS) and nitric oxide (NO), increased activation of ERK1/2 and enhanced β-amyloid neurotoxic effects [101, 102].

In contrast, another study demonstrated that elevated S100B levels could have a beneficial role in neurons via activation of PI3K/Akt and NF-kB [103]. In astrocytes, overstimulation of iNOS leads to an increase in NO, which in turn causes astrocyte death by apoptosis [104]. Moreover, high S100B stimulates IL-1β expression and release of IL-6 and TNF-α from astrocytes, meaning that S100B is likely to take part on activation of the brain inflammatory response [105]. Conversely, high S100B may be beneficial in the course of brain inflammatory processes, once induced apoptosis is suggested to contribute to the reduction of activated astrocytes [105]. At micromolar levels, S100B activates microglia and in combination with cofactors like bacterial endotoxin or IFN-γ upregulate iNOS expression and NO release from microglia [17]. Activation of microglia in the presence of high levels of S100B is evidenced by NF-kB and AP-1-dependent stimulation of cytokine expression and cyclooxygenase-2 (COX-2) expression [106].

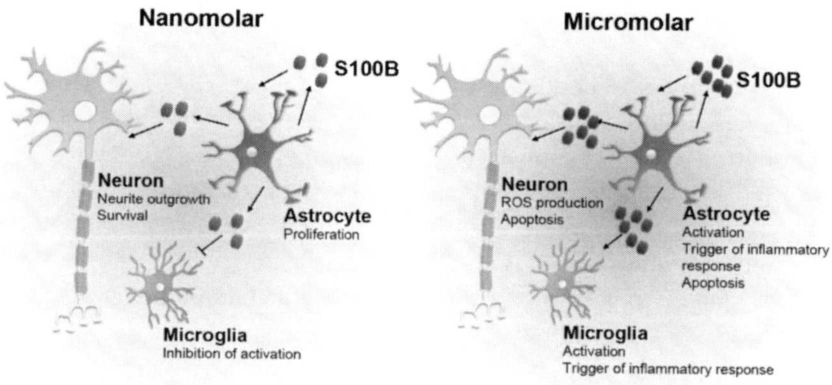

Figure 1. Schematic representation of S100B extracellular effects in neurons, astrocytes and microglia. At nanomolar concentrations S100B exerts a beneficial effect on central nervous system cells, inducing neurite outgrowth, neuronal survival, astrocyte proliferation and inhibition of microglia activation. In contrast, higher concentrations (macromolar levels), usually released upon injury, are detrimental, favouring a proinflammatory scenery with astrocyte and microglial reactivity and neuron apoptosis.

3.3. Role of S100B on Oligodendrogenesis

Regarding oligodendrocytes, little is known about the S100B effects in their development and maturation. Nevertheless, it has been described that

S100B is a marker of terminal differentiation for oligodendrocyte populations of the mouse embryonic hindbrain and spinal cord, being the S100B expression in these populations comparable to that of astrocytes [56]. However, S100B is also transiently expressed in the nuclei of oligodendroglial progenitor cells committed to differentiate into mature oligodendrocytes and its expression persists in slow diving adult oligodendrocyte progenitor cells and preoligodendrocytes [5]. Moreover, S100B expression starts in myelinating oligodendrocytes after birth and reaches high postnatal levels in mature myelinating oligodendrocytes (Figure 2) [56]. The dual localization of S100B in oligodendrocytes suggests that this protein is involved in cytoplasmic and nuclear Ca^{2+}/Zn^{2+}-dependent cell regulation processes. Previous data have also suggested that S100B modulates oligodendrocyte maturation but the mechanism is not yet understood. So, although absence of S100B seems not to have any effect on the number of oligodendrocyte progenitor cells that developed from primary glial cultures or multipotent neurospheres, it causes delay in morphological and phenotypic markers associated with oligodendrocyte maturation in oligodendrocyte progenitor cells derived from $S100B^{-/-}$ mice [5]. In addition, the increase in S100B expression during the transition from non-myelinating to myelinating cells, when elaboration of myelin sheaths occurs concomitantly with a drastic loss of arborisation, suggests that S100B could have a role in the regulation of oligodendrocyte cell shape, as already demonstrated for neuronal cells. This S100B role is consistent with its association with microtubular structures in cultured oligodendrocytes [16]. In fact, oligodendrocytes express microtubule-associated protein 2 and tau [107], whose phosphorylation by protein kinase II is inhibited *in vitro* in a Ca^{2+}-dependent manner by S100B [108]. S100B also participates in the signaling cascade controlling neurofilament phosphorylation and axon calibre [109], a function of oligodendrocytes that seems to be uncoupled from myelination [110], through its association and inhibition of PKA-dependent phosphorylation of the large isoform of the myelin-associated glycoprotein [111]. A recent study identified mitochondrial ATAD3A protein as the major high-affinity S100B target protein in oligodendrocyte progenitor cells [112]. ATAD3A is anchored into the mitochondrial inner membrane, mainly at sites that may form contacts with the outer membrane, and regulates mitochondrial dynamics and diverse cell responses, ranging from mitochondrial metabolism, cell growth and mitochondrial fission [113]. So, it has been proposed that S100B could assist ATAD3A protein during cytoplasmatic processing by preventing aggregation and facilitating its subcellular localization at the mitochondria [112]. So, since oligodendrocyte precursor cell differentiation requires *de novo* mitochondrial protein synthesis, this study suggests that ATAD3A is required for a proper cell growth and differentiation.

Regarding the effects of extracellular S100B on oligodendrocytes, there are no reports concerning the deleterious action that increased levels of S100B may have in their development. Our recent studies have demonstrated that exposure to high levels of S100B during proliferation leads to oligodendrocyte differentiation impairment, with a significant reduction of mature oligodendrocytes and an increase in oligodendrocyte progenitor cells. In addition, high doses of S100B are also able to induce oligodendrocyte maturation arrest and marked impairment of both chemotaxis and chemokinesis (Figure 2).

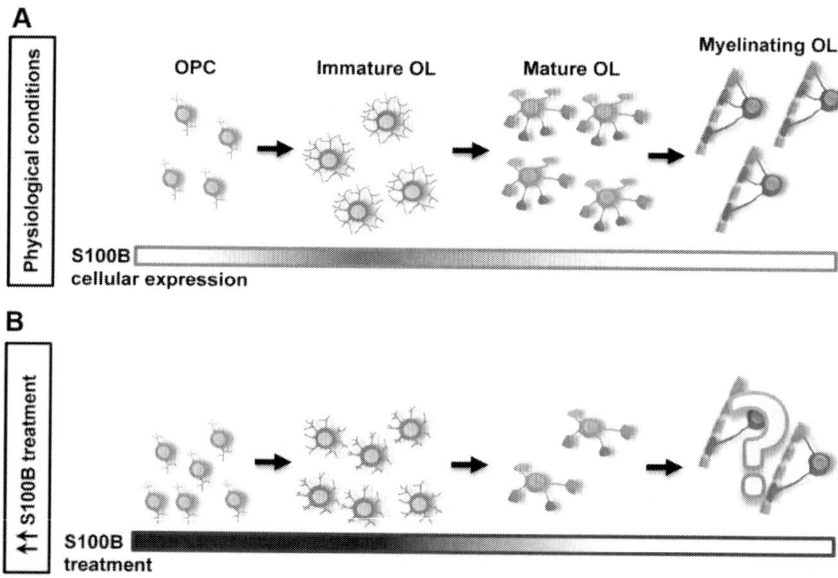

Figure 2. S100B and oligodendrocyte development. Schematic representation of (A) S100B expression along oligodendrocyte (OL) lineage progression and (B) effects of high S100B levels in OL development. In OL primary cultures, treatment with high S100B doses during proliferation or initial differentiation impairs OL differentiation leading to an increase in oligodendrocyte precursor cells (OPC) and a decrease in mature OL. Also, morphological maturation of mature OL is delayed with increased number of OL poorly branched and decreased OL with complex branched processes and OL that partially form myelin-related membranes.

Moreover, S100B can indirectly lead to oligodendrocyte death. Due to oligodendrocyte high metabolic rate, elevated intracellular iron, low concentration of the antioxidative glutathione and expression of α-amino-3-hydroxy-5-methyl-4-isoxazolepropionic acid (AMPA), kainate and N-methyl-D-aspartate receptor (NMDA) receptors, oligodendrocytes are particularly susceptible to oxidative damage and mitochondrial injury, as well as to excitotoxic cell death and to inflammatory cytokines [114].

Taking all this concepts together, extracellular S100B is now being used as glial marker, being considered a parameter of glial activation or commitment in several situations of brain injury, namely in myelin-related disorders.

4. S100B As a Biomarker

Biomarkers are defined as a laboratory measurement that reflects the activity of a disease process, providing diagnostic or prognostic value in a determined altered physiological condition or disease state [115]. The search for specific peripheral biochemical markers of brain tissue activity and injury has increased over the last decade. In this context, since S100B is primarily produced by astrocytes in the CNS, intra- and extracellular mRNA and protein levels have been used as putative markers of astrocyte activation and/or death in a variety of brain injury conditions [116, 117]. S100B is elevated and released into the circulation in several CNS disorders, including perinatal brain distress, traumatic brain damage, acute brain injury, brain ischemia, brain tumours, neuroinflammatory/neurodegenerative diseases and psychiatric disorders. In fact, some studies correlate S100B variations with neuroimaging alterations, intracerebral pressure measurements and neurological signals [118]. Although in many instances its release may be an effect of the condition rather than the cause, experimental findings point to S100B as a possible biomarker of CNS injury, as well as an important therapeutic target. Nonetheless, it may be noted the existence of controversial aspects regarding the use of S100B as a marker of brain damage, since several biochemical features of this protein and its physiological and pathological variations are not well characterized. The significance of serum S100B variations is often unknown and debatable due to the possible extra cerebral sources of S100B or methodological problems surrounding its measurement. Indeed, it should be noted that immunoassays and mRNA quantification have characterized other cells as S100B-expressing cells, particularly adipocytes, chondrocytes, lymphocytes, bone marrow cells and melanoma cells, which can contribute to the serum S100B content [119-122].

4.1. Measurement of S100B Levels

The S100B protein was detected for the first time, in extracellular biological fluids, in the CSF of patients with multiple sclerosis (MS) [123]. Since then, research on the role of S100B as a biomarker of brain distress has been extended to other biological fluids including blood plasma [124], cord blood [125], amniotic fluid [126], urine [126] and saliva [127]. It is noteworthy that S100B is also present in human milk at higher amount than the one in CSF, blood or urine [128]. Besides the biological fluids, S100B can also be detected in brain tissue as that of patients with Alzheimer's disease and Down's syndrome (DS) [129].

Several methods have been developed to determine S100B levels in serum and CSF with high sensitivity, such as radioimmune assays, immunoradiometric assays, luminescence immunoassays, enzyme immunoassays, fluoroimmune assays, enzyme-linked immunosorbent assays, electrochemiluminescence assays, high performance liquid chromatography, optic immunization, mass spectroscopy, western blot, and quantitative polymerase chain reaction (PCR) [130, 131].

All these methods differ on specificity, sensitivity, sample application and economic costs. In fact, the most recent immunoassays are more simple, sensitive and less expensive. However, the commercially available S100B diagnostic kit must be more carefully used due to possible cross reactivity with other S100 proteins co-expressed in the brain [20].

5. S100B Association with Myelin-Related Disorders

The increase of S100B levels in the brain has been associated with numerous disorders with altered myelination, such as DS, schizophrenia, mood disorders, spinocerebellar ataxia type 3 (SCA3), Guillain-Barré syndrome (GBS) and MS.

Table 2. S100B in myelin-related disorders

Condition/disorder	Serum	CSF	*Post-mortem* tissue	Oligodendrocyte/myelin alterations
Down's Syndrome	Increased S100B levels in foetuses blood [126, 138, 139, 249, 250] and adult patients blood [137][136]	-	Increased S100B expression in temporal lobe [129, 140] and hippocampus [251] Increased expression in activated astrocytes in neocortex of fetal, young and adult patients [141] Expression of S100B in astrocytes increases with advancing gestation age [142]	Increased Olig2 expression in foetal frontal cortices [146] and temporal lobe [147] No changes in myelination in foetuses [145] but postnatal delay in myelination is observed in newborns, infants and children [145] Decreased expression of CNPase oligodendrocyte marker in frontal and temporal cortex [148]
Schizophrenia	Increased S100B levels in patients with chronic schizophrenia, in acute relapses and in first-episode [156-159, 252-255]	Increased S100B levels in schizophrenia patients in acute episodes of relapse [159, 161]	Higher number of S100B+ glia in cortical brain regions [162]	Lower S100B+ oligodendrocyte number patients with residual schizophrenia [162] Less mature oligodendrocytes in corpus callosum [163] and decreased number of oligodendrocytes [152, 256-258] Decreased expression of Olig2 and myelin proteins [153, 154, 259] Myelin abnormalities [150, 151, 260, 261], including myelin sheath lamellae damage and alterations in oligodendrocyte mitochondria and their apoptosis [155]
Mood disorders	Increased S100B levels in patients with major depressive disorder and bipolar disorder [165, 179, 180, 183]	Increased S100B levels in acute episodes of major depressive disorder [184]	Changes in S100B in lateral prefrontal and parietal cortices in bipolar disorder [186]	Decreased density of S100B+ oligodendrocytes in the left alveus in bipolar disorder [188] Lower number of oligodendrocytes in anterior cingulate cortex, orbitofrontal cortex, dorsolateral prefrontal cortex, amygdala and hippocampus [152, 155, 176, 177, 262]

Table 2. (Continued)

Condition/disorder	Serum	CSF	*Post-mortem* tissue	Oligodendrocyte/myelin alterations
Mood disorders	Higher S100B levels in elderly patients when compared with young patients [181]		Increased density of S100B+ astrocytes in the hippocampus CA1 pyramidal layer in major depressive disorder and bipolar disorder [188]	Changes in white matter connectivity between unipolar and bipolar depression [178]
Spinocerebellar ataxia type 3	No differences in S100B levels [195] Increased S100B levels [196]	-	-	Decreased number of myelinated fibres and myelin thickness [194] Peripheral demyelination [194]
Guillain-Barré syndrome	-	Correlation of S100B levels with months to recovery [202] Increased S100B levels on admission [203]	-	Myelin sheath damage and consequent demyelination in acute inflammatory demyelinating polyneuropathy [200, 263] Swelling and fragmentation of myelin from nerve roots [201] Macrophages filled with large amounts of myelin [201]
Multiple sclerosis	Increased S100B levels within the first seven days after the beginning of exacerbation [218] Increased S100B levels [7]	Increased S100B levels, especially in the acute phase of exacerbation [123, 215] Increased S100B levels [7] No significant difference was found between multiple sclerosis types [217]	Increased S100B levels in white and grey matter [7] Increased S100B expression in the lesion area in active and chronic active demyelinating lesions S100B+ cells are mainly astrocytes	Focal demyelination [210]

In recent years, several *in vitro* and *in vivo* animal experiments regarding brain damage and neurodegeneration have been conducted in order to clarify the potential of S100B in brain damage. Studies with animal models presenting high levels of S100B revealed behavioural changes, together with structural and morphological characteristics similar to those that occur in some brain pathologies [132, 133].

Notwithstanding the mechanism by which S100B performs all its functions is yet not fully elucidated. However, as described before it is known that deleterious role of S100B is probably related to their ability to act as a cytokine, being involved in the inflammatory response associated with brain damage, to stimulate ROS and NO production and to activate microglia.

Major findings of S100B on the pathophysiology of myelin-related disorders are summarized in Table 2.

5.1. Down's Syndrome

DS is the most common chromosome abnormality, associated with mental retardation and neurological abnormalities followed by precocious neurodegeneration and early onset of Alzheimer's disease [134]. The primary cause of DS is currently attributed to ongoing neuronal degeneration due to the presence of an extra copy of chromosome 21 (HSA21), the one where S100B is found. The triplicated chromosome in DS leads to lifelong overexpression of the respective encoded genes, although it is not fully clear how this condition leads to the syndrome phenotype. However, it is thought that several pathological changes observed in DS, like decreased neuronal and glial cell numbers and delayed myelination, are related to S100B overexpression. In addition to the increased levels of S100B, myelination defects observed in DS can also be related with delayed oligodendrocyte maturation since the transcription factor Olig2, which plays a crucial role in oligodendrocyte maturation, is encoded by a gene located also on chromosome 21 [135].

It was reported a higher immunocontent of S100B in DS patients when compared with control patients, whereas serum levels in DS were not age-related as it is observed in normal individuals [136]. Another study showed that the relative DNA level and quantity of S100B were higher in the blood of DS subjects than those observed in the control group [137]. Also, preliminary findings demonstrated increased S100B levels in DS foetuses blood [138] and amniotic fluid when compared with matched controls [139], as expected in cases of gene triplication.

Post-mortem brain studies of patients with DS demonstrated increased S100B expression [129, 140] and S100B+ cells through all ages [141]. Interestingly, the DS brain contains more S100B than the respective controls, when evaluated after birth [142]. Similarly, Marks et al., showed a raise in S100B mRNA and protein levels in the cerebellum of patients with DS between 1 and 18 months of age, but with no differences in the rates of accumulation between DS and normal subjects [116]. Additionally, the expression of S100B correlates positively with cerebral cortical β-amyloid deposition and, at the same time, the number of S100B-positive astrocytes showed a positive correlation with the numeric density of β-amyloid plaques and β-amyloid precursor protein (βAPP) overexpression [140, 141]. Genomic and functional studies profiling human DS neural progenitors revealed a constitutive overexpression of HSA21 associated S100B, which *per si* led to increased ROS formation and activation of stress response kinases, resulting in a compensatory aquaporin 4 expression [143]. Further, HSA21 associated S100B and βAPP levels are simultaneously increased in DS human neural progenitors and the overexpression of these proteins disrupt mitochondrial membrane potentials and redox states, leading to mitochondrial dysfunction and apoptosis in a dose-dependent manner. The ongoing neural injury and inflammation through both βAPP and S100B overexpression further promotes a gliocentric human neural progenitors phenotype, which coincides with a decline in neurogenesis [144]. In addition, taking into account the deleterious effects of increased S100B levels in oligodendrocytes, changes in oligodendrogenesis and myelination observed in DS can be related with S100B levels. In this disease, although myelination is not affected in DS foetuses and newborns, myelin formation is delayed postnatally for up to 12 months in infants with 2 months-6 years [145].

In addition, impaired proliferation of neural progenitors in the ventricular zone is related with increased Olig2 expression in DS foetal frontal cortices when compared with age-matched controls [146]. The altered pattern of Olig2 expression suggests a role in abnormal myelin formation in DS brains. Indeed, a recent study suggested that the increased number of Olig2+ cells in the temporal lobe white matter is probably related to an increase in immature oligodendrocytes [147]. Another study also detected that 2',3'-cyclic-nucleotide 3'-phosphodiesterase (CNPase), a myelin-associated enzyme, was significantly decreased in frontal and temporal cortex of DS patients, reflecting decreased oligodendroglial density and/or reduced myelination [148].

5.2. Schizophrenia

Schizophrenia is the most common psychotic illness, being considered a severe psychiatric disorder that presents several symptoms including hallucinations, disorganized speech/thinking and cognitive dysfunction [149]. Although most studies on schizophrenic brain defects have focused on alterations in neurons and grey matter, more recent reports also showed alterations in white matter. Indeed, specific abnormalities in myelin are increasingly observed in patients with schizophrenia [150, 151], including decreased number of oligodendrocytes [152], lower expression of Olig2 and myelin proteins [153, 154], damaged myelin sheath lamellae, irregularities in oligodendrocyte mitochondria and cell death by apoptosis [155]. These oligodendrocyte and myelin changes could be, at least in part, due to the increased S100B levels found in schizophrenic patients.

The great majority of the research regarding the association of schizophrenia to S100B was performed in serum. The first published study showed that serum S100B concentration is significantly increased in schizophrenic patients when compared to controls [156]. After that, several authors have found increased S100B levels in patients with chronic schizophrenia, in acute relapses and in first-episode compared to healthy controls [157, 158]. Most authors report no sex differences in S100B levels in patients with schizophrenia [159]. However, a recent study showed increased levels of S100B in the serum of schizophrenic female patients, but not in males [160].

Regarding CSF, only a few studies reported increased concentrations of S100B in the CSF of schizophrenic patients during acute episodes of relapse [159, 161]. In accordance, Steiner et al., [161] reported the existence of increased S100B concentrations in CSF and serum of acute first-onset schizophrenic patients, but no differences in the concentrations of GFAP, myelin basic protein and neuron-specific enolase.

In post-mortem tissue, only the study of Steiner et al., [162] indicated the existence of more S100B-immunopositive glia in cortical brain regions of schizophrenic patients. These authors described the presence of lower S100B+ oligodendrocyte count in the subgroup of patients with residual schizophrenia [162]. In addition, it was described the downregulation of S100B in the nuclear proteome of the corpus callosum from schizophrenic patients when compared to mentally healthy controls [163]. So, as corpus callosum is essentially composed by white matter, this study suggests that S100B has a potential role in the control of oligodendrocyte maturation. Indeed, mature oligodendrocytes present higher cytoplasmic content of S100B, while immature oligodendrocytes display higher nuclear S100B expression [5]. So, the diminished expression of S100B in the nuclear proteome in the corpus callosum [163] may indicate that less oligodendrocytes are maturating in schizophrenia brains.

5.3. Mood Disorders

Mood disorders, comprising major depressive disorder (MDD) and bipolar disorder (BD), usually show very often marked changes in neuroplasticity and glial response [164, 165]. Patients with MDD differ considerably in their course of illness: most patients have recurrent episodes, but others suffer only one single depressive episode during their lifetime [166]. MDD is among the most common forms of psychiatric disease with a worldwide prevalence of 16% across the lifespan and 6.6% across a 12-month period [167]. BD is a chronic and disabling disorder characterized by impairments in social, emotional and academic functioning in childhood and early adolescence [168]. Moreover, the prevalence rate of bipolar spectrum disorder has been estimated to be 2% among children and adolescents in the community [169].

Histopathological post-mortem studies have shown that glia density is reduced in several brain regions, such as anterior cingulate cortex, orbitofrontal cortex, dorsolateral prefrontal cortex and hippocampus in association with reduced prefrontal grey matter [170-172]. It is thought that hippocampus has an important role in these diseases due to its key function in both emotional and cognitive aspects of mood disorders [173]. Changes in these regions are attributed mainly to astrocytes [174, 175] and oligodendrocytes [176], namely in those located in amygdala [177]. Diffusion tensor imaging revealed significant differences in the white matter connectivity between unipolar and bipolar depression, predominantly in the left hemisphere, which is an important finding for clinical practice [178].

The hypothesis that S100B plays an important role in the pathophysiology of mood disorders is based on several studies demonstrating increased S100B levels in the serum of patients suffering MDD and BD [179, 180], what corroborates the glial involvement in the pathogenesis of mood disorders. In addition, S100B concentration is higher in elderly subjects in comparison with young subjects with mood disorders [181]. Increased serum S100B levels have been observed in two rat models of depression, as well [182]. If these disorders are mainly glial disorders, as suggested by Rajkowska [170], it should be expected elevated S100B serum levels in parallel with unaltered level of neuronal marker protein neuron specific enolase. In fact, in depressive patients at admission and discharge, S100B concentrations are higher when compared to control subjects, while neuron specific enolase is not different between these patients and control subjects for both time points [183]. Regarding CSF S100B concentrations, only a few studies tried to establish a relationship between these levels and MDD, but the results are controversial. The only study performed in human samples showed increased S100B levels in acute episodes of MDD [184]. However, in an animal model of depression, it was described the presence of reduced S100B levels [185].

In post-mortem tissue, the levels of S100B are altered in the lateral prefrontal and parietal cortices in BD, with a decrease in Brodmann's area 9 and increase in Brodmann's area 40 [186]. Studies in animal models revealed decreased S100B protein content in prefrontal regions [182] and in the hippocampus [187]. Recently, Gos et al., [162] showed bilateral increase of the density of S100B+ astrocytes in the CA1 pyramidal layer of the hippocampus from MDD and BD patients, while only BD patients revealed a decreased density of S100B+ oligodendrocytes in the left alveus [188]. These changes in oligodendrocyte density can be explained by disturbances in oligodendrocyte maturation leading to a decrease in immature S100B+ pre-oligodendrocytes, as well as by damage or dysfunction of oligodendrocytes. Alterations in glial S100B expression in the hippocampus seem to be specific of mood disorders because no significant changes were observed in S100B+ glia in hippocampal subregions of schizophrenic patients.

5.4. Spinocerebellar Ataxia type 3 (Machado-Joseph Disease)

SCA3, also known as Machado-Joseph disease, is an autosomal dominant neurodegenerative disorder caused by expansion of CAG trinucleotide repeats in the chromosomal locus 14q24.3-q31 region [189]. In addition, it was revealed that the early onset and the progressively severe nature of the clinical features were correlated with the number of CAG repeat size [190]. This trinucleotide CAG repeat encodes an elongated polyglutamine tract with the *ataxin-3* gene [189]. Histopathological studies have disclosed that there are extensive neuronal cell loss and gliosis in cerebellum, basal ganglia, brainstem, Clarke's columns, dentate nucleus, pontine nuclei and substantia nigra, together with aggregates of the pathogenic ataxin-3 in neuronal nuclei and cytoplasm, as well as in axons of the affected fibre tracts [191]. The pathophysiology of SCA3 is due to neuropathy at the dorsal root ganglia [192], and moderate reduction in the nerve conduction velocity [193], which may indicate abnormalities in Schwann cells, the myelinating cells of the peripheral nervous system. In fact, the involvement of Schwann cells in the neuropathy of SCA3 was already reported [194]. Recently, Suga et al., [194] showed a decrease in the number of myelinated fibrer and in myelin thickness, together with axonal sprouting in the post mortem sural nerves from SCA3. The authors showed an accumulation of intracytoplasmatic aggregates of the pathogenic ataxin-3 in Schwann cells, which may be related with the peripheral demyelination observed in SCA3.

Regarding the S100B role in this disease, Tort et al., [195] have investigated S100B serum concentrations in SCA3 patients. The S100B levels of these subjects were not statistically different comparing with controls. Moreover, S100B levels were moderately correlated with disease duration and depression score, but no relationship was observed with molecular parameters or clinical evaluation. Notwithstanding, in a more recent study it was found higher S100B concentrations in SCA3 patients compared with the healthy controls [196]. The same work also showed no correlation between the CAG repeat size and the S100B levels in different age groups of SCA3 patients, which may indicate that the CAG repeats do not affect S100B production or release. So, further work will be needed to clarify the S100B role in this disease.

5.5. Guillain-Barré Syndrome

GBS, an acute immune-mediated inflammatory polyneuropathy, is the most common cause of acute neuromuscular paralysis [197]. Up to one-third of GBS patients require mechanical ventilation, approximately 20% of hospitalized patients may have a long-term disability, and acute mortality remains relatively high [198, 199]. The most common subtypes of GBS are the acute inflammatory demyelinating polyneuropathy (AIDP) and the acute motor axonal neuropathy (AMAN) [197]. AIDP is characterized by an autoimmune response against Schwann cells, and consequent demyelination, whereas AMAN is caused by autoimmune response against peripheral axons that leads to axonal degeneration [197]. In more detail, during AIDP, blood macrophages invade the peripheral nervous system and target antigens on Schwann cells or myelin sheath with the help of cytokines released from activated T lymphocytes and activated macrophages, destroying the myelin sheaths [200]. On the other hand, in AMAN diseases it is indicated that macrophages invade the Ranvier nodes, causing damage or dysfunction of the axons and the surrounding Schwann cells leaving the myelin sheath intact [201]. Overall, in GBS, myelin from nerve roots suffers swelling and fragmentation, which are then phagocytosed by macrophages becoming filled with large amounts of myelin [201].

The first study about S100B in the CSF of GBS patients demonstrated a significant correlation of CSF content in S100B with the duration of recovery, indicating that this protein may be of prognostic relevance in GBS [202]. In addition, a prospective multicenter study showed significantly higher CSF S100B levels in GBS patients on admission compared with control subjects [203]. A recent study proved that the CSF S100B levels at the acute phase positively correlate with the clinical severity of AIDP rather than AMAN, suggesting potential usefulness in assessing AIDP prognosis [204]. Such S100B values were not higher in patients with AIDP than in patients with AMAN, which is possible related with S100B release from Schwann cells and myelin sheath after demyelination that occurs not only in AIDP but also in AMAN. In addition, Piazza et al., [205] have similarly reported increased S100B levels in GBS patients.

5.5. Multiple Sclerosis

MS, an inflammatory, demyelinating disease of the CNS with associated neurodegeneration [206], is the most common chronic neurological disease among young adults, with a mean age of onset of approximately 30 years and a prevalence of 1.3/1000 people in the developed world [207]. The onset of the disease is characterized by episodes or relapses of common symptoms, like impaired vision and deficits in sensation [208]. At later stages patients can present severe disabilities including paralysis, incontinence and cognitive impairment, involving memory loss and concentration problems [209]. Full recovery from initial relapses usually occurs during the early stages of the disease course, but after a variable period of relapsing-remitting phase (RRMS) a progressive build-up of residual neurological dysfunction develops along the secondary progressive phase (SPMS). However, approximately 10 to 20% of the individuals with MS show a progressive disease since the onset, with no relapse or remission episodes, termed primary progressive MS (PPMS). The most obvious pathological finding in MS brain tissue is focal demyelination, which may affect any part of the CNS [210]. Although demyelination has long been considered a marked feature of MS, axonal damage and neuronal loss are likewise accepted as consequences of the disease and showed to be correlated with its progression and permanent neurologic disability [211]. In fact, some studies proposed that axonal impairment occurs in areas of active inflammatory demyelination and in an early phase of the disease course [212, 213]. Moreover, microglia can also release toxic molecules such as proteases and nitrogen species leading to oligodendrocyte injury and demyelination [214].

S100B levels can also have an important role in MS. Michetti et al., [123] reported increased S100 concentration in the CSF of patients with MS, especially during the acute phase of exacerbation. Later, a subsequent study with MS patients through 5 weeks following the onset of an acute exacerbation revealed a maximal S100B expression in the third week, which decreased thereafter [215]. However, no changes were found in S100B CSF concentrations at various stages of disease in another study [216]. More recently, Petzold et al., [7] reported significantly higher CSF S100B levels in MS patients when compared with controls. Lately, although S100B increased levels were found in CSF and serum of patients with MS, no significant difference was found between MS types [217]. A recent study of our group has shown that S100B levels are elevated in the CSF and serum of RRMS patients at the time of diagnosis (personal communication). Missler et al., [218] reported that plasma concentrations were significantly elevated in MS patients within the first seven days after the beginning of MS exacerbation [218]. Furthermore, it was described a substantial trend for increasing S100B levels from PPMS to SPMS to RRMS, whereas the highest S100B levels were observed in the RRMS patients [7]. Moreover, in the same study pointed to a correlation between S100B level and 9HPT, a brief, standardized, quantitative test of upper extremity function in PPMS patients.

The only post-mortem published study on S100B expression in MS showed elevated levels of this protein in the white matter (subacute plaques), as well as in grey matter (cortical zone) of MS patients compared with control subjects [7]. Our recent data in post-mortem material of MS patients showed increased expression of S100B and its receptor RAGE in the lesion area, in active demyelinating MS lesions, while chronic active lesions displayed increased S100B in demyelinated areas with lower expression of RAGE in the rim. Reactive astrocytes were identified as the predominant cellular source of S100B, whereas RAGE was expressed by activated microglia/macrophages. Using an experimental demyelinating model we have also demonstrated that demyelination induces a marked upregulation and release of S100B protein, in parallel with astrocytosis, microgliosis and enhanced gene expression of key proinflammatory cytokines and inflammasome-related molecules.

All these evidences suggest that S100B might have a role in the development of MS and corresponding features.

6. Anti-S100B Therapies in Myelin-Related Disorders

Considering all the evidences about the S100B increase in numerous diseases and its toxic effects, it can be assumed that its inhibition may have a beneficial outcome, suggesting S100B as an emerging therapeutic target. In fact, a series of inhibitors for S100B, like pentamidine and chlorpromazine, were discovered for treating malignant melanoma [219, 220]. The pentamidine inhibits S100B-mediated effects because of its ability to disrupt S100B-p53 interaction, reducing significantly cell growth [63, 65, 221]. In addition, several studies demonstrated that pentamidine have also anti-inflammatory properties [222-225]. Interestingly, a recent study in an animal model of Alzheimer's disease showed that pentamidine reduces S100B and its receptor RAGE expression, induces p53 expression in astrocytes and reduces the expression of proinflammatory mediators and markers, such as GFAP, iNOS, cyclooxygenase 2 and p-p38, in the hippocampus [226]. However, one of the limiting factors of pentamidine resides in its low blood-brain barrier crossing, being necessary new pharmacokinetic approaches to increase its delivery into the brain. Vig et al., [227] have recently reported that TRTK12, a S100B inhibitory peptide, modulates Purkinje cell morphology in slice cultures and improves behavioural abnormalities in an animal model of spinocerebellar ataxia. S100B effects can additionally be modulated by inhibition of its binding to RAGE using specific antibodies or small molecules [228]. However, RAGE is not the unique receptor that mediates S100B effects. So, it seems more appropriate to inhibit the protein itself. In this context, our recent findings demonstrated that in an *ex vivo* model of demyelination, the neutralization of S100B using a specific antibody prevents demyelination and astrocyte reactivity, while reducing the expression of proinflammatory and inflammasome-related mediators. Alternative therapeutic strategies that may be used to control S100B expression are based on the regulation of gene products, via gene therapy approaches, or regulation of S100B protein action through inhibitory binding to specific aptamers [229]. Future studies are needed to investigate the best strategy and its advantages in animal models of disorders that present increased S100B levels.

Conclusion

S100 proteins are Ca^{2+}-sensor proteins that present an important role in the regulation of several functions, such as cell proliferation and differentiation, cell morphology, cell motility, protein phosphorylation, enzymatic activity, intracellular Ca^{2+} homeostasis, apoptosis, transcription and inflammatory response. In particular, S100B, which is mainly expressed by astrocytes in the brain, exerts a proliferative function at intracellular level, while extracellular effects depend upon its concentration. Indeed, S100B promote cell proliferation and differentiation for nanomolar concentrations, but cellular death for micromolar levels. In this context, S100B is considered a marker of brain damage since it is able to cross the blood-brain barrier and its levels can be easily detected in serum and/or CSF. Most attractive is the role of S100B on oligodendrogenesis and its potential implication in myelin-related disorders. In fact, multiple studies demonstrated increased S100B levels in CSF and/or serum in several diseases that show marked oligodendrocyte/ myelin changes, including DS, schizophrenia, mood disorders, SCA3, GBS and MS. However, regulation of S100B expression requires more investigation and for its usage as therapeutic tool it will be necessary the identification of highly specific inhibitors and their assays in *in vivo* studies.

References

[1] Moore, B.W., A soluble protein characteristic of the nervous system. *Biochem Biophys Res Commun*, 1965. 19(6): p. 739-44.

[2] Donato, R., B.R. Cannon, G. Sorci, F. Riuzzi, K. Hsu, D.J. Weber, and C.L. Geczy, Functions of S100 proteins. *Curr Mol Med,* 2013. 13(1): p. 24-57.

[3] Yardan, T., A.K. Erenler, A. Baydin, K. Aydin, and C. Cokluk, Usefulness of S100B protein in neurological disorders. *J Pak Med Assoc,* 2011. 61(3): p. 276-81.

[4] Sorci, G., R. Bianchi, F. Riuzzi, C. Tubaro, C. Arcuri, I. Giambanco, and R. Donato, S100B Protein, A Damage-Associated Molecular Pattern

Protein in the Brain and Heart, and Beyond. *Cardiovasc Psychiatry Neurol,* 2010. 656481.
[5] Deloulme, J.C., E. Raponi, B.J. Gentil, N. Bertacchi, A. Marks, G. Labourdette, and J. Baudier, Nuclear expression of S100B in oligodendrocyte progenitor cells correlates with differentiation toward the oligodendroglial lineage and modulates oligodendrocytes maturation. *Mol Cell Neurosci,* 2004. 27(4): p. 453-65.
[6] Steiner, J., H.G. Bernstein, B. Bogerts, T. Gos, C. Richter-Landsberg, M.T. Wunderlich, and G. Keilhoff, S100B is expressed in, and released from, OLN-93 oligodendrocytes: Influence of serum and glucose deprivation. *Neuroscience*, 2008. 154(2): p. 496-503.
[7] Petzold, A., M.J. Eikelenboom, D. Gveric, G. Keir, M. Chapman, R.H. Lazeron, M.L. Cuzner, C.H. Polman, B.M. Uitdehaag, E.J. Thompson, and G. Giovannoni, Markers for different glial cell responses in multiple sclerosis: clinical and pathological correlations. *Brain*, 2002. 125(Pt 7): p. 1462-73.
[8] Marenholz, I., C.W. Heizmann, and G. Fritz, S100 proteins in mouse and man: from evolution to function and pathology (including an update of the nomenclature). *Biochem Biophys Res Commun*, 2004. 322(4): p. 1111-22.
[9] Donato, R., S-100 proteins. *Cell Calcium,* 1986. 7(3): p. 123-45.
[10] Schafer, B.W., J.M. Fritschy, P. Murmann, H. Troxler, I. Durussel, C.W. Heizmann, and J.A. Cox, Brain S100A5 is a novel calcium-, zinc-, and copper ion-binding protein of the EF-hand superfamily. *J Biol Chem,* 2000. 275(39): p. 30623-30.
[11] Donato, R., S100: a multigenic family of calcium-modulated proteins of the EF-hand type with intracellular and extracellular functional roles. *Int J Biochem Cell Biol,* 2001. 33(7): p. 637-68.
[12] Krieg, P., M. Schuppler, R. Koesters, A. Mincheva, P. Lichter, and F. Marks, Repetin (Rptn), a new member of the "fused gene" subgroup within the S100 gene family encoding a murine epidermal differentiation protein. *Genomics,* 1997. 43(3): p. 339-48.
[13] Presland, R.B., J.A. Bassuk, J.R. Kimball, and B.A. Dale, Characterization of two distinct calcium-binding sites in the amino-terminus of human profilaggrin. *J Invest Dermatol*, 1995. 104(2): p. 218-23.
[14] Fritz, G., H.M. Botelho, L.A. Morozova-Roche, and C.M. Gomes, Natural and amyloid self-assembly of S100 proteins: structural basis of functional diversity. *FEBS J,* 2010. 277(22): p. 4578-90.

[15] Smith, S.P. and G.S. Shaw, A novel calcium-sensitive switch revealed by the structure of human S100B in the calcium-bound form. *Structure,* 1998. 6(2): p. 211-22.

[16] Richter-Landsberg, C. and M. Heinrich, S-100 immunoreactivity in rat brain glial cultures is associated with both astrocytes and oligodendrocytes. *J Neurosci Res,* 1995. 42(5): p. 657-65.

[17] Adami, C., G. Sorci, E. Blasi, A.L. Agneletti, F. Bistoni, and R. Donato, S100B expression in and effects on microglia. *Glia,* 2001. 33(2): p. 131-42.

[18] Schafer, B.W. and C.W. Heizmann, The S100 family of EF-hand calcium-binding proteins: functions and pathology. *Trends Biochem Sci,* 1996. 21(4): p. 134-40.

[19] Donato, R., Intracellular and extracellular roles of S100 proteins. *Microsc Res Tech*, 2003. 60(6): p. 540-51.

[20] Heizmann, C.W., G. Fritz, and B.W. Schafer, S100 proteins: structure, functions and pathology. *Front Biosci*, 2002. 7: p. d1356-68.

[21] Schwaller, B., Cytosolic Ca2+ buffers. *Cold Spring Harb Perspect Biol*, 2010. 2(11): a004051.

[22] Zimmer, D.B. and D.J. Weber, The Calcium-Dependent Interaction of S100B with Its Protein Targets. *Cardiovasc Psychiatry Neurol*, 2010. 728052.

[23] Santamaria-Kisiel, L., A.C. Rintala-Dempsey, and G.S. Shaw, Calcium-dependent and -independent interactions of the S100 protein family. *Biochem J,* 2006. 396(2): p. 201-14.

[24] Chazin, W.J., Relating form and function of EF-hand calcium binding proteins. *Acc Chem Res*, 2011. 44(3): p. 171-9.

[25] Zolese, G., A. Tangorra, G. Curatola, I. Giambanco, and R. Donato, Interaction of S-100b protein with cardiolipin vesicles as monitored by electron spin resonance, pyrene fluorescence and circular dichroism. *Cell Calcium,* 1988. 9(3): p. 149-57.

[26] Urban, C.F., D. Ermert, M. Schmid, U. Abu-Abed, C. Goosmann, W. Nacken, V. Brinkmann, P.R. Jungblut, and A. Zychlinsky, Neutrophil extracellular traps contain calprotectin, a cytosolic protein complex involved in host defense against Candida albicans. *PLoS Pathog,* 2009. 5(10): e1000639.

[27] Donato, R., Functional roles of S100 proteins, calcium-binding proteins of the EF-hand type. *Biochim Biophys Acta,* 1999. 1450(3): p. 191-231.

[28] Donato, R., RAGE: a single receptor for several ligands and different cellular responses: the case of certain S100 proteins. *Curr Mol Med,* 2007. 7(8): p. 711-24.

[29] Leclerc, E., G. Fritz, S.W. Vetter, and C.W. Heizmann, Binding of S100 proteins to RAGE: an update. *Biochim Biophys Acta*, 2009. 1793(6): p. 993-1007.

[30] Rezvanpour, A. and G.S. Shaw, Unique S100 target protein interactions. *Gen Physiol Biophys*, 2009. 28 Focus Issue: p. F39-46.

[31] Yan, W.X., C. Armishaw, J. Goyette, Z. Yang, H. Cai, P. Alewood, and C.L. Geczy, Mast cell and monocyte recruitment by S100A12 and its hinge domain. *J Biol Chem*, 2008. 283(19): p. 13035-43.

[32] Donato, R., G. Sorci, F. Riuzzi, C. Arcuri, R. Bianchi, F. Brozzi, C. Tubaro, and I. Giambanco, S100B's double life: intracellular regulator and extracellular signal. *Biochim Biophys Acta*, 2009. 1793(6): p. 1008-22.

[33] Isobe, T., N. Ishioka, T. Masuda, Y. Takahashi, S. Ganno, and T. Okuyama, A rapid separation of S100 subunits by high performance liquid chromatography: the subunit compositions of S100 proteins. *Biochem Int*, 1983. 6(3): p. 419-26.

[34] Leclerc, E. and C.W. Heizmann, The importance of Ca2+/Zn2+ signaling S100 proteins and RAGE in translational medicine. *Front Biosci* (Schol Ed), 2011. 3: p. 1232-62.

[35] Markowitz, J., R.R. Rustandi, K.M. Varney, P.T. Wilder, R. Udan, S.L. Wu, W.D. Horrocks, and D.J. Weber, Calcium-binding properties of wild-type and EF-hand mutants of S100B in the presence and absence of a peptide derived from the C-terminal negative regulatory domain of p53. *Biochemistry*, 2005. 44(19): p. 7305-14.

[36] Drohat, A.C., D.M. Baldisseri, R.R. Rustandi, and D.J. Weber, Solution structure of calcium-bound rat S100B(betabeta) as determined by nuclear magnetic resonance spectroscopy. *Biochemistry*, 1998. 37(9): p. 2729-40.

[37] Drohat, A.C., J.C. Amburgey, F. Abildgaard, M.R. Starich, D. Baldisseri, and D.J. Weber, Solution structure of rat apo-S100B(beta beta) as determined by NMR spectroscopy. *Biochemistry,* 1996. 35(36): p. 11577-88.

[38] Wilder, P.T., K.M. Varney, M.B. Weiss, R.K. Gitti, and D.J. Weber, Solution structure of zinc- and calcium-bound rat S100B as determined by nuclear magnetic resonance spectroscopy. *Biochemistry,* 2005. 44(15): p. 5690-702.

[39] McClintock, K.A. and G.S. Shaw, A novel S100 target conformation is revealed by the solution structure of the Ca2+-S100B-TRTK-12 complex. *J Biol Chem,* 2003. 278(8): p. 6251-7.

[40] Rustandi, R.R., D.M. Baldisseri, and D.J. Weber, Structure of the negative regulatory domain of p53 bound to S100B(betabeta). *Nat Struct Biol,* 2000. 7(7): p. 570-4.

[41] Drohat, A.C., E. Nenortas, D. Beckett, and D.J. Weber, Oligomerization state of S100B at nanomolar concentration determined by large-zone analytical gel filtration chromatography. *Protein Sci,* 1997. 6(7): p. 1577-82.

[42] Thulin, E., T. Kesvatera, and S. Linse, Molecular determinants of S100B oligomer formation. *PLoS One,* 2011. 6(3): e14768.

[43] Van Eldik, L.J. and D.B. Zimmer, Secretion of S-100 from rat C6 glioma cells. *Brain Res,* 1987. 436(2): p. 367-70.

[44] Ciccarelli, R., P. Di Iorio, V. Bruno, G. Battaglia, I. D'Alimonte, M. D'Onofrio, F. Nicoletti, and F. Caciagli, Activation of A(1) adenosine or mGlu3 metabotropic glutamate receptors enhances the release of nerve growth factor and S-100beta protein from cultured astrocytes. *Glia,* 1999. 27(3): p. 275-81.

[45] Edwards, M.M. and S.R. Robinson, TNF alpha affects the expression of GFAP and S100B: implications for Alzheimer's disease. *J Neural Transm,* 2006. 113(11): p. 1709-15.

[46] Zimmer, D.B., E.H. Cornwall, A. Landar, and W. Song, The S100 protein family: history, function, and expression. *Brain Res Bull,* 1995. 37(4): p. 417-29.

[47] Halonen, S.K., T. Woods, K. McInnerney, and L.M. Weiss, Microarray analysis of IFN-gamma response genes in astrocytes. *J Neuroimmunol,* 2006. 175(1-2): p. 19-30.

[48] Arcuri, C., I. Giambanco, R. Bianchi, and R. Donato, Annexin V, annexin VI, S100A1 and S100B in developing and adult avian skeletal muscles. *Neuroscience,* 2002. 109(2): p. 371-88.

[49] Rothermundt, M., M. Peters, J.H. Prehn, and V. Arolt, S100B in brain damage and neurodegeneration. *Microsc Res Tech,* 2003. 60(6): p. 614-32.

[50] Michetti, F., V. Corvino, M.C. Geloso, W. Lattanzi, C. Bernardini, L. Serpero, and D. Gazzolo, The S100B protein in biological fluids: more than a lifelong biomarker of brain distress. *J Neurochem,* 2012. 120(5): p. 644-59.

[51] Ahlemeyer, B., H. Beier, I. Semkova, C. Schaper, and J. Krieglstein, S-100beta protects cultured neurons against glutamate- and staurosporine-induced damage and is involved in the antiapoptotic action of the 5 HT(1A)-receptor agonist, Bay x 3702. *Brain Res*, 2000. 858(1): p. 121-8.

[52] Nishi, M., M. Kawata, and E.C. Azmitia, Trophic interactions between brain-derived neurotrophic factor and s100beta on cultured serotonergic neurons. *Brain Res,* 2000. 868(1): p. 113-8.

[53] Nishiyama, H., T. Knopfel, S. Endo, and S. Itohara, Glial protein S100B modulates long-term neuronal synaptic plasticity. *Proc Natl Acad Sci USA*, 2002. 99(6): p. 4037-42.

[54] Koppal, T., A.G. Lam, L. Guo, and L.J. Van Eldik, S100B proteins that lack one or both cysteine residues can induce inflammatory responses in astrocytes and microglia. *Neurochem Int*, 2001. 39(5-6): p. 401-7.

[55] Sorci, G., F. Riuzzi, C. Arcuri, C. Tubaro, R. Bianchi, I. Giambanco, and R. Donato, S100B protein in tissue development, repair and regeneration. *World J Biol Chem*, 2013. 4(1): p. 1-12.

[56] Hachem, S., A. Aguirre, V. Vives, A. Marks, V. Gallo, and C. Legraverend, Spatial and temporal expression of S100B in cells of oligodendrocyte lineage. *Glia*, 2005. 51(2): p. 81-97.

[57] Steiner, J., H.G. Bernstein, H. Bielau, A. Berndt, R. Brisch, C. Mawrin, G. Keilhoff, and B. Bogerts, Evidence for a wide extra-astrocytic distribution of S100B in human brain. *BMC Neurosci*, 2007. 8:2.

[58] Rosenberg, S.S. and N.C. Spitzer, Calcium signaling in neuronal development. *Cold Spring Harb Perspect Biol*, 2011. 3(10): a004259.

[59] Deitmer, J.W., A.J. Verkhratsky, and C. Lohr, Calcium signalling in glial cells. *Cell Calcium*, 1998. 24(5-6): p. 405-16.

[60] Salama, I., P.S. Malone, F. Mihaimeed, and J.L. Jones, A review of the S100 proteins in cancer. *Eur J Surg Oncol*, 2008. 34(4): p. 357-64.

[61] Tamaskovic, R., S.J. Bichsel, H. Rogniaux, M.R. Stegert, and B.A. Hemmings, Mechanism of Ca2+-mediated regulation of NDR protein kinase through autophosphorylation and phosphorylation by an upstream kinase. *J Biol Chem,* 2003. 278(9): p. 6710-8.

[62] Lin, J., M. Blake, C. Tang, D. Zimmer, R.R. Rustandi, D.J. Weber, and F. Carrier, Inhibition of p53 transcriptional activity by the S100B calcium-binding protein. *J Biol Chem*, 2001. 276(37): p. 35037-41.

[63] Markowitz, J., I. Chen, R. Gitti, D.M. Baldisseri, Y. Pan, R. Udan, F. Carrier, A.D. MacKerell, Jr., and D.J. Weber, Identification and characterization of small molecule inhibitors of the calcium-dependent

S100B-p53 tumor suppressor interaction. *J Med Chem*, 2004. 47(21): p. 5085-93.

[64] Brozzi, F., C. Arcuri, I. Giambanco, and R. Donato, S100B Protein Regulates Astrocyte Shape and Migration via Interaction with Src Kinase: Implications for Astrocyte Development, Activation, and Tumor Growth. *J Biol Chem*, 2009. 284(13): p. 8797-811.

[65] Arcuri, C., R. Bianchi, F. Brozzi, and R. Donato, S100B increases proliferation in PC12 neuronal cells and reduces their responsiveness to nerve growth factor via Akt activation. *J Biol Chem,* 2005. 280(6): p. 4402-14.

[66] Raponi, E., F. Agenes, C. Delphin, N. Assard, J. Baudier, C. Legraverend, and J.C. Deloulme, S100B expression defines a state in which GFAP-expressing cells lose their neural stem cell potential and acquire a more mature developmental stage. *Glia,* 2007. 55(2): p. 165-77.

[67] Sahoo, N., J. Troger, S.H. Heinemann, and R. Schonherr, Current inhibition of human EAG1 potassium channels by the Ca2+ binding protein S100B. *FEBS Lett,* 2010. 584(18): p. 3896-900.

[68] Donato, R., Calcium-independent, pH-regulated effects of S-100 proteins on assembly-disassembly of brain microtubule protein in vitro. *J Biol Chem,* 1988. 263(1): p. 106-10.

[69] Sorci, G., A.L. Agneletti, and R. Donato, Effects of S100A1 and S100B on microtubule stability. An in vitro study using triton-cytoskeletons from astrocyte and myoblast cell lines. *Neuroscience,* 2000. 99(4): p. 773-83.

[70] Davey, G.E., P. Murmann, and C.W. Heizmann, Intracellular Ca2+ and Zn2+ levels regulate the alternative cell density-dependent secretion of S100B in human glioblastoma cells. *J Biol Chem*, 2001. 276(33): p. 30819-26.

[71] Garbuglia, M., M. Verzini, and R. Donato, Annexin VI binds S100A1 and S100B and blocks the ability of S100A1 and S100B to inhibit desmin and GFAP assemblies into intermediate filaments. *Cell Calcium,* 1998. 24(3): p. 177-91.

[72] Sorci, G., A.L. Agneletti, R. Bianchi, and R. Donato, Association of S100B with intermediate filaments and microtubules in glial cells. *Biochim Biophys Acta*, 1998. 1448(2): p. 277-89.

[73] Hai, C.M. and Z. Gu, Caldesmon phosphorylation in actin cytoskeletal remodeling. *Eur J Cell Biol*, 2006. 85(3-4): p. 305-9.

[74] Skripnikova, E.V. and N.B. Gusev, Interaction of smooth muscle caldesmon with S-100 protein. *FEBS Lett,* 1989. 257(2): p. 380-2.

[75] Mbele, G.O., J.C. Deloulme, B.J. Gentil, C. Delphin, M. Ferro, J. Garin, M. Takahashi, and J. Baudier, The zinc- and calcium-binding S100B interacts and co-localizes with IQGAP1 during dynamic rearrangement of cell membranes. *J Biol Chem*, 2002. 277(51): p. 49998-50007.

[76] Watanabe, T., S. Wang, J. Noritake, K. Sato, M. Fukata, M. Takefuji, M. Nakagawa, N. Izumi, T. Akiyama, and K. Kaibuchi, Interaction with IQGAP1 links APC to Rac1, Cdc42, and actin filaments during cell polarization and migration. *Dev Cell*, 2004. 7(6): p. 871-83.

[77] Landar, A., G. Caddell, J. Chessher, and D.B. Zimmer, Identification of an S100A1/S100B target protein: phosphoglucomutase. *Cell Calcium*, 1996. 20(3): p. 279-85.

[78] Sen, J. and A. Belli, S100B in neuropathologic states: the CRP of the brain? *J Neurosci Res,* 2007. 85(7): p. 1373-80.

[79] Rambotti, M.G., I. Giambanco, A. Spreca, and R. Donato, S100B and S100A1 proteins in bovine retina:their calcium-dependent stimulation of a membrane-bound guanylate cyclase activity as investigated by ultracytochemistry. *Neuroscience*, 1999. 92(3): p. 1089-101.

[80] Pozdnyakov, N., A. Margulis, and A. Sitaramayya, Identification of effector binding sites on S100 beta: studies with guanylate cyclase and p80, a retinal phosphoprotein. *Biochemistry,* 1998. 37(30): p. 10701-8.

[81] Liu, Y., D.C. Buck, and K.A. Neve, Novel interaction of the dopamine D2 receptor and the Ca2+ binding protein S100B: role in D2 receptor function. *Mol Pharmacol,* 2008. 74(2): p. 371-8.

[82] Ohta, K., S. Kuno, I. Mizuta, A. Fujinami, H. Matsui, and M. Ohta, Effects of dopamine agonists bromocriptine, pergolide, cabergoline, and SKF-38393 on GDNF, NGF, and BDNF synthesis in cultured mouse astrocytes. *Life Sci,* 2003. 73(5): p. 617-26.

[83] Li, A., H. Guo, X. Luo, J. Sheng, S. Yang, Y. Yin, J. Zhou, and J. Zhou, Apomorphine-induced activation of dopamine receptors modulates FGF-2 expression in astrocytic cultures and promotes survival of dopaminergic neurons. *FASEB J,* 2006. 20(8): p. 1263-5.

[84] Shashoua, V.E., G.W. Hesse, and B.W. Moore, Proteins of the brain extracellular fluid: evidence for release of S-100 protein. *J Neurochem,* 1984. 42(6): p. 1536-41.

[85] de Souza, D.F., M.C. Leite, A. Quincozes-Santos, P. Nardin, L.S. Tortorelli, M.M. Rigo, C. Gottfried, R.B. Leal, and C.A. Goncalves, S100B secretion is stimulated by IL-1beta in glial cultures and

hippocampal slices of rats: Likely involvement of MAPK pathway. *J Neuroimmunol*, 2009. 206(1-2): p. 52-7.
[86] Goncalves, D., J. Karl, M. Leite, L. Rotta, C. Salbego, E. Rocha, S. Wofchuk, and C.A. Goncalves, High glutamate decreases S100B secretion stimulated by serum deprivation in astrocytes. *Neuroreport,* 2002. 13(12): p. 1533-5.
[87] Nardin, P., F. Tramontina, M.C. Leite, A.C. Tramontina, A. Quincozes-Santos, L.M. de Almeida, A.M. Battastini, C. Gottfried, and C.A. Goncalves, S100B content and secretion decrease in astrocytes cultured in high-glucose medium. *Neurochem Int,* 2007. 50(5): p. 774-82.
[88] Reddy, M.A., S.L. Li, S. Sahar, Y.S. Kim, Z.G. Xu, L. Lanting, and R. Natarajan, Key role of Src kinase in S100B-induced activation of the receptor for advanced glycation end products in vascular smooth muscle cells. *J Biol Chem*, 2006. 281(19): p. 13685-93.
[89] Leite, M.C., F. Galland, D.F. de Souza, M.C. Guerra, L. Bobermin, R. Biasibetti, C. Gottfried, and C.A. Goncalves, Gap junction inhibitors modulate S100B secretion in astrocyte cultures and acute hippocampal slices. *J Neurosci Res,* 2009. 87(11): p. 2439-46.
[90] Neeper, M., A.M. Schmidt, J. Brett, S.D. Yan, F. Wang, Y.C. Pan, K. Elliston, D. Stern, and A. Shaw, Cloning and expression of a cell surface receptor for advanced glycosylation end products of proteins. *J Biol Chem,* 1992. 267(21): p. 14998-5004.
[91] Gupta, A.A., R.H. Chou, H. Li, L.W. Yang, and C. Yu, Structural insights into the interaction of human S100B and basic fibroblast growth factor (FGF2): Effects on FGFR1 receptor signaling. *Biochim Biophys Acta,* 2013. 1834(12): p. 2606-19.
[92] Riuzzi, F., G. Sorci, and R. Donato, S100B protein regulates myoblast proliferation and differentiation by activating FGFR1 in a bFGF-dependent manner. *J Cell Sci,* 2011. 124(Pt 14): p. 2389-400.
[93] Kleindienst, A., M.J. McGinn, H.B. Harvey, R.J. Colello, R.J. Hamm, and M.R. Bullock, Enhanced hippocampal neurogenesis by intraventricular S100B infusion is associated with improved cognitive recovery after traumatic brain injury. *J Neurotrauma*, 2005. 22(6): p. 645-55.
[94] Kogel, D., M. Peters, H.G. Konig, S.M. Hashemi, N.T. Bui, V. Arolt, M. Rothermundt, and J.H. Prehn, S100B potently activates p65/c-Rel transcriptional complexes in hippocampal neurons: Clinical implications for the role of S100B in excitotoxic brain injury. *Neuroscience*, 2004. 127(4): p. 913-20.

[95] Tramontina, F., A.C. Tramontina, D.F. Souza, M.C. Leite, C. Gottfried, D.O. Souza, S.T. Wofchuk, and C.A. Goncalves, Glutamate uptake is stimulated by extracellular S100B in hippocampal astrocytes. *Cell Mol Neurobiol,* 2006. 26(1): p. 81-6.

[96] Reali, C., F. Scintu, R. Pillai, R. Donato, F. Michetti, and V. Sogos, S100b counteracts effects of the neurotoxicant trimethyltin on astrocytes and microglia. *J Neurosci Res,* 2005. 81(5): p. 677-86.

[97] Hu, J., F. Castets, J.L. Guevara, and L.J. Van Eldik, S100 beta stimulates inducible nitric oxide synthase activity and mRNA levels in rat cortical astrocytes. *J Biol Chem,* 1996. 271(5): p. 2543-7.

[98] Lam, A.G., T. Koppal, K.T. Akama, L. Guo, J.M. Craft, B. Samy, J.P. Schavocky, D.M. Watterson, and L.J. Van Eldik, Mechanism of glial activation by S100B: involvement of the transcription factor NFkappaB. *Neurobiol Aging,* 2001. 22(5): p. 765-72.

[99] Gonçalves, D.S., G. Lenz, J. Karl, C.A. Goncalves, and R. Rodnight, Extracellular S100B protein modulates ERK in astrocyte cultures. *Neuroreport,* 2000. 11(4): p. 807-9.

[100] Zhang, L., W. Liu, D. Alizadeh, D. Zhao, O. Farrukh, J. Lin, S.A. Badie, and B. Badie, S100B attenuates microglia activation in gliomas: possible role of STAT3 pathway. *Glia,* 2011. 59(3): p. 486-98.

[101] Hu, J., A. Ferreira, and L.J. Van Eldik, S100beta induces neuronal cell death through nitric oxide release from astrocytes. *J Neurochem*, 1997. 69(6): p. 2294-301.

[102] Businaro, R., S. Leone, C. Fabrizi, G. Sorci, R. Donato, G.M. Lauro, and L. Fumagalli, S100B protects LAN-5 neuroblastoma cells against Abeta amyloid-induced neurotoxicity via RAGE engagement at low doses but increases Abeta amyloid neurotoxicity at high doses. *J Neurosci Res,* 2006. 83(5): p. 897-906.

[103] Leclerc, E., G. Fritz, M. Weibel, C.W. Heizmann, and A. Galichet, S100B and S100A6 differentially modulate cell survival by interacting with distinct RAGE (receptor for advanced glycation end products) immunoglobulin domains. *J Biol Chem,* 2007. 282(43): p. 31317-31.

[104] Hu, J. and L.J. Van Eldik, S100 beta induces apoptotic cell death in cultured astrocytes via a nitric oxide-dependent pathway. *Biochim Biophys Acta,* 1996. 1313(3): p. 239-45.

[105] Ponath, G., C. Schettler, F. Kaestner, B. Voigt, D. Wentker, V. Arolt, and M. Rothermundt, Autocrine S100B effects on astrocytes are mediated via RAGE. *J Neuroimmunol*, 2007. 184(1-2): p. 214-22.

[106] Bianchi, R., I. Giambanco, and R. Donato, S100B/RAGE-dependent activation of microglia via NF-kappaB and AP-1 Co-regulation of COX-2 expression by S100B, IL-1beta and TNF-alpha. *Neurobiol Aging*, 2010. 31(4): p. 665-77.

[107] LoPresti, P., Regulation and differential expression of tau mRNA isoforms as oligodendrocytes mature in vivo: implications for myelination. *Glia,* 2002. 37(3): p. 250-7.

[108] Baudier, J. and R.D. Cole, Interactions between the microtubule-associated tau proteins and S100b regulate tau phosphorylation by the Ca2+/calmodulin-dependent protein kinase II. *J Biol Chem*, 1988. 263(12): p. 5876-83.

[109] Dashiell, S.M., S.L. Tanner, H.C. Pant, and R.H. Quarles, Myelin-associated glycoprotein modulates expression and phosphorylation of neuronal cytoskeletal elements and their associated kinases. *J Neurochem,* 2002. 81(6): p. 1263-72.

[110] Lappe-Siefke, C., S. Goebbels, M. Gravel, E. Nicksch, J. Lee, P.E. Braun, I.R. Griffiths, and K.A. Nave, Disruption of Cnp1 uncouples oligodendroglial functions in axonal support and myelination. *Nat Genet,* 2003. 33(3): p. 366-74.

[111] Kursula, P., V.P. Lehto, and A.M. Heape, S100beta inhibits the phosphorylation of the L-MAG cytoplasmic domain by PKA. *Brain Res Mol Brain Res*, 2000. 76(2): p. 407-10.

[112] Gilquin, B., B.R. Cannon, A. Hubstenberger, B. Moulouel, E. Falk, N. Merle, N. Assard, S. Kieffer, D. Rousseau, P.T. Wilder, D.J. Weber, and J. Baudier, The calcium-dependent interaction between S100B and the mitochondrial AAA ATPase ATAD3A and the role of this complex in the cytoplasmic processing of ATAD3A. *Mol Cell Biol,* 2010. 30(11): p. 2724-36.

[113] Gilquin, B., E. Taillebourg, N. Cherradi, A. Hubstenberger, O. Gay, N. Merle, N. Assard, M.O. Fauvarque, S. Tomohiro, O. Kuge, and J. Baudier, The AAA+ ATPase ATAD3A controls mitochondrial dynamics at the interface of the inner and outer membranes. *Mol Cell Biol,* 2010. 30(8): p. 1984-96.

[114] Back, S.A. and P.A. Rosenberg, Pathophysiology of glia in perinatal white matter injury. *Glia,* 2014. 62(11): p. 1790-815.

[115] Katz, R., Biomarkers and surrogate markers: an FDA perspective. *NeuroRx*, 2004. 1(2): p. 189-95.

[116] Marks, A., D. O'Hanlon, M. Lei, M.E. Percy, and L.E. Becker, Accumulation of S100 beta mRNA and protein in cerebellum during

infancy in Down syndrome and control subjects. *Brain Res Mol Brain Res,* 1996. 36(2): p. 343-8.

[117] Kleindienst, A. and M. Ross Bullock, A critical analysis of the role of the neurotrophic protein S100B in acute brain injury. *J Neurotrauma,* 2006. 23(8): p. 1185-200.

[118] Bloomfield, S.M., J. McKinney, L. Smith, and J. Brisman, Reliability of S100B in predicting severity of central nervous system injury. *Neurocrit Care*, 2007. 6(2): p. 121-38.

[119] Gonçalves, C.A., M.C. Leite, and M.C. Guerra, Adipocytes as an Important Source of Serum S100B and Possible Roles of This Protein in Adipose Tissue. *Cardiovasc Psychiatry Neurol,* 2010. 2010:790431.

[120] Steiner, J., N. Marquardt, I. Pauls, K. Schiltz, H. Rahmoune, S. Bahn, B. Bogerts, R.E. Schmidt, and R. Jacobs, Human CD8(+) T cells and NK cells express and secrete S100B upon stimulation. *Brain Behav Immun,* 2011. 25(6): p. 1233-41.

[121] Diaz-Romero, J., A. Quintin, E. Schoenholzer, C. Pauli, A. Despont, M.A. Zumstein, S. Kohl, and D. Nesic, S100A1 and S100B expression patterns identify differentiation status of human articular chondrocytes. *J Cell Physiol*, 2014. 229(8): p. 1106-17.

[122] Leclerc, E., C.W. Heizmann, and S.W. Vetter, RAGE and S100 protein transcription levels are highly variable in human melanoma tumors and cells. *Gen Physiol Biophys,* 2009. 28 Focus Issue: p. F65-75.

[123] Michetti, F., A. Massaro, and M. Murazio, The nervous system-specific S-100 antigen in cerebrospinal fluid of multiple sclerosis patients. *Neurosci Lett,* 1979. 11(2): p. 171-5.

[124] Kato, K., S. Kimura, R. Semba, F. Suzuki, and T. Nakajima, Increase in S-100 protein levels in blood plasma by epinephrine. *J Biochem*, 1983. 94(3): p. 1009-11.

[125] Gazzolo, D., P. Vinesi, E. Marinoni, R. Di Iorio, M. Marras, M. Lituania, P. Bruschettini, and F. Michetti, S100B protein concentrations in cord blood: correlations with gestational age in term and preterm deliveries. *Clin Chem*, 2000. 46(7): p. 998-1000.

[126] Gazzolo, D., M. Bruschettini, V. Corvino, R. Oliva, R. Sarli, M. Lituania, P. Bruschettini, and F. Michetti, S100b protein concentrations in amniotic fluid correlate with gestational age and with cerebral ultrasound scanning results in healthy fetuses. *Clin Chem*, 2001. 47(5): p. 954-6.

[127] Gazzolo, D., M. Lituania, M. Bruschettini, S. Ciotti, R. Sacchi, G. Serra, M.G. Calevo, V. Corvino, G. Buonocore, and F. Michetti, S100B protein

levels in saliva: correlation with gestational age in normal term and preterm newborns. *Clin Biochem,* 2005. 38(3): p. 229-33.

[128] Galvano, F., A. Frigiola, L. Gagliardi, S. Ciotti, M. Bognanno, A.M. Iacopino, F. Nigro, G.L. Tina, D. Cavallaro, M. Mussap, A. Piva, E. Grilli, F. Michetti, and D. Gazzolo, S100B milk concentration in mammalian species. *Front Biosci* (Elite Ed), 2009. 1: p. 542-6.

[129] Griffin, W.S., L.C. Stanley, C. Ling, L. White, V. MacLeod, L.J. Perrot, C.L. White, 3rd, and C. Araoz, Brain interleukin 1 and S-100 immunoreactivity are elevated in Down syndrome and Alzheimer disease. *Proc Natl Acad Sci USA,* 1989. 86(19): p. 7611-5.

[130] Heizmann, C.W., S100B protein in clinical diagnostics: assay specificity. *Clin Chem*, 2004. 50(1): p. 249-51.

[131] Smit, L.H., C.M. Korse, and J.M. Bonfrer, Comparison of four different assays for determination of serum S-100B. *Int J Biol Markers*, 2005. 20(1): p. 34-42.

[132] Mori, T., N. Koyama, G.W. Arendash, Y. Horikoshi-Sakuraba, J. Tan, and T. Town, Overexpression of human S100B exacerbates cerebral amyloidosis and gliosis in the Tg2576 mouse model of Alzheimer's disease. *Glia,* 2010. 58(3): p. 300-14.

[133] Bell, K., D. Shokrian, C. Potenzieri, and P.M. Whitaker-Azmitia, Harm avoidance, anxiety, and response to novelty in the adolescent S-100beta transgenic mouse: role of serotonin and relevance to Down syndrome. *Neuropsychopharmacology*, 2003. 28(10): p. 1810-6.

[134] Engidawork, E. and G. Lubec, Protein expression in Down syndrome brain. *Amino Acids*, 2001. 21(4): p. 331-61.

[135] Maire, C.L., A. Wegener, C. Kerninon, and B. Nait Oumesmar, Gain-of-function of Olig transcription factors enhances oligodendrogenesis and myelination. *Stem Cells*, 2010. 28(9): p. 1611-22.

[136] Netto, C.B., I.R. Siqueira, C. Fochesatto, L.V. Portela, M. da Purificacao Tavares, D.O. Souza, R. Giugliani, and C.A. Goncalves, S100B content and SOD activity in amniotic fluid of pregnancies with Down syndrome. *Clin Biochem*, 2004. 37(2): p. 134-7.

[137] Yang, Y.H., M.S. Nam, and E.S. Yang, Rapid prenatal diagnosis of trisomy 21 by real-time quantitative polymerase chain reaction with amplification of small tandem repeats and S100B in chromosome 21. Yonsei Med J, 2005. 46(2): p. 193-7.

[138] Abraha, H.D., P.L. Noble, K.H. Nicolaides, and R.A. Sherwood, Maternal serum S100 protein in normal and Down syndrome pregnancies. *Prenat Diagn*, 1999. 19(4): p. 334-6.

[139] Tort, A.B., L.V. Portela, M. da Purificacao Tavares, C.A. Goncalves, C. Netto, R. Giugliani, and D.O. Souza, Specificity and sensitivity of S100B levels in amniotic fluid for Down syndrome diagnosis. *Life Sci,* 2004. 76(4): p. 379-84.

[140] Royston, M.C., J.E. McKenzie, S.M. Gentleman, J.G. Sheng, D.M. Mann, W.S. Griffin, and R.E. Mrak, Overexpression of s100beta in Down's syndrome: correlation with patient age and with beta-amyloid deposition. *Neuropathol Appl Neurobiol*, 1999. 25(5): p. 387-93.

[141] Griffin, W.S., J.G. Sheng, J.E. McKenzie, M.C. Royston, S.M. Gentleman, R.A. Brumback, L.C. Cork, M.R. Del Bigio, G.W. Roberts, and R.E. Mrak, Life-long overexpression of S100beta in Down's syndrome: implications for Alzheimer pathogenesis. *Neurobiol Aging*, 1998. 19(5): p. 401-5.

[142] Tiu, S.C., W.Y. Chan, C.W. Heizmann, B.W. Schafer, S.Y. Shu, and D.T. Yew, Differential expression of S100B and S100A6(1) in the human fetal and aged cerebral cortex. *Brain Res Dev Brain Res*, 2000. 119(2): p. 159-68.

[143] Esposito, G., J. Imitola, J. Lu, D. De Filippis, C. Scuderi, V.S. Ganesh, R. Folkerth, J. Hecht, S. Shin, T. Iuvone, J. Chesnut, L. Steardo, and V. Sheen, Genomic and functional profiling of human Down syndrome neural progenitors implicates S100B and aquaporin 4 in cell injury. *Hum Mol Genet,* 2008. 17(3): p. 440-57.

[144] Lu, J., G. Esposito, C. Scuderi, L. Steardo, L.C. Delli-Bovi, J.L. Hecht, B.C. Dickinson, C.J. Chang, T. Mori, and V. Sheen, S100B and APP promote a gliocentric shift and impaired neurogenesis in Down syndrome neural progenitors. *PLoS One,* 2011. 6(7): p. e22126.

[145] Wisniewski, K.E. and B. Schmidt-Sidor, Postnatal delay of myelin formation in brains from Down syndrome infants and children. *Clin Neuropathol,* 1989. 8(2): p. 55-62.

[146] Lu, J., G. Lian, H. Zhou, G. Esposito, L. Steardo, L.C. Delli-Bovi, J.L. Hecht, Q.R. Lu, and V. Sheen, OLIG2 over-expression impairs proliferation of human Down syndrome neural progenitors. *Hum Mol Genet,* 2012. 21(10): p. 2330-40.

[147] Kanaumi, T., I. Milenkovic, H. Adle-Biassette, E. Aronica, and G.G. Kovacs, Non-neuronal cell responses differ between normal and Down syndrome developing brains. *Int J Dev Neurosci*, 2013. 31(8): p. 796-803.

[148] Vlkolinsky, R., N. Cairns, M. Fountoulakis, and G. Lubec, Decreased brain levels of 2',3'-cyclic nucleotide-3'-phosphodiesterase in Down

syndrome and Alzheimer's disease. Neurobiol Aging, 2001. 22(4): p. 547-53.
[149] McGrath, J., S. Saha, D. Chant, and J. Welham, Schizophrenia: a concise overview of incidence, prevalence, and mortality. *Epidemiol Rev*, 2008. 30: p. 67-76.
[150] Takahashi, N., T. Sakurai, K.L. Davis, and J.D. Buxbaum, Linking oligodendrocyte and myelin dysfunction to neurocircuitry abnormalities in schizophrenia. *Prog Neurobiol*, 2011. 93(1): p. 13-24.
[151] Kyriakopoulos, M. and S. Frangou, Recent diffusion tensor imaging findings in early stages of schizophrenia. *Curr Opin Psychiatry*, 2009. 22(2): p. 168-76.
[152] Uranova, N.A., V.M. Vostrikov, D.D. Orlovskaya, and V.I. Rachmanova, Oligodendroglial density in the prefrontal cortex in schizophrenia and mood disorders: a study from the Stanley *Neuropathology Consortium. Schizophr Res*, 2004. 67(2-3): p. 269-75.
[153] Hakak, Y., J.R. Walker, C. Li, W.H. Wong, K.L. Davis, J.D. Buxbaum, V. Haroutunian, and A.A. Fienberg, Genome-wide expression analysis reveals dysregulation of myelination-related genes in chronic schizophrenia. *Proc Natl Acad Sci USA,* 2001. 98(8): p. 4746-51.
[154] Matthews, P.R., S.L. Eastwood, and P.J. Harrison, Reduced myelin basic protein and actin-related gene expression in visual cortex in schizophrenia. *PLoS One*, 2012. 7(6): p. e38211.
[155] Uranova, N., D. Orlovskaya, O. Vikhreva, I. Zimina, N. Kolomeets, V. Vostrikov, and V. Rachmanova, Electron microscopy of oligodendroglia in severe mental illness. Brain Res Bull, 2001. 55(5): p. 597-610.
[156] Wiesmann, M., K.P. Wandinger, U. Missler, D. Eckhoff, M. Rothermundt, V. Arolt, and H. Kirchner, Elevated plasma levels of S-100b protein in schizophrenic patients. *Biol Psychiatry*, 1999. 45(11): p. 1508-11.
[157] Zhang, X.Y., M.H. Xiu, C. Song, C. Chen da, G.Y. Wu, C.N. Haile, T.A. Kosten, and T.R. Kosten, Increased serum S100B in never-medicated and medicated schizophrenic patients. *J Psychiatr Res*, 2010. 44(16): p. 1236-40.
[158] Schroeter, M.L., H. Abdul-Khaliq, S. Fruhauf, R. Hohne, G. Schick, A. Diefenbacher, and I.E. Blasig, Serum S100B is increased during early treatment with antipsychotics and in deficit schizophrenia. *Schizophr Res,* 2003. 62(3): p. 231-6.
[159] Rothermundt, M., G. Ponath, T. Glaser, G. Hetzel, and V. Arolt, S100B serum levels and long-term improvement of negative symptoms in

patients with schizophrenia. *Neuropsychopharmacology*, 2004. 29(5): p. 1004-11.

[160] O'Connell, K., J. Thakore, and K.K. Dev, Levels of S100B are raised in female patients with schizophrenia. *BMC Psychiatry*, 2013. 13: 146.

[161] Steiner, J., H. Bielau, H.G. Bernstein, B. Bogerts, and M.T. Wunderlich, Increased cerebrospinal fluid and serum levels of S100B in first-onset schizophrenia are not related to a degenerative release of glial fibrillar acidic protein, myelin basic protein and neurone-specific enolase from glia or neurones. *J Neurol Neurosurg Psychiatry*, 2006. 77(11): p. 1284-7.

[162] Steiner, J., H.G. Bernstein, H. Bielau, N. Farkas, J. Winter, H. Dobrowolny, R. Brisch, T. Gos, C. Mawrin, A.M. Myint, and B. Bogerts, S100B-immunopositive glia is elevated in paranoid as compared to residual schizophrenia: a morphometric study. *J Psychiatr Res,* 2008. 42(10): p. 868-76.

[163] Steiner, J., A. Schmitt, M.L. Schroeter, B. Bogerts, P. Falkai, C.W. Turck, and D. Martins-de-Souza, S100B is downregulated in the nuclear proteome of schizophrenia corpus callosum. *Eur Arch Psychiatry Clin Neurosci,* 2014. 264(4): p. 311-6.

[164] Manji, H.K., G.J. Moore, G. Rajkowska, and G. Chen, Neuroplasticity and cellular resilience in mood disorders. *Mol Psychiatry*, 2000. 5(6): p. 578-93.

[165] Schroeter, M.L., H. Abdul-Khaliq, J. Sacher, J. Steiner, I.E. Blasig, and K. Mueller, Mood disorders are glial disorders: evidence from in vivo studies. *Cardiovasc Psychiatry Neurol*, 2010. 2010:780645.

[166] Hardeveld, F., J. Spijker, R. De Graaf, W.A. Nolen, and A.T. Beekman, Prevalence and predictors of recurrence of major depressive disorder in the adult population. *Acta Psychiatr Scand*, 2010. 122(3): p. 184-91.

[167] Kessler, R.C., P. Berglund, O. Demler, R. Jin, D. Koretz, K.R. Merikangas, A.J. Rush, E.E. Walters, P.S. Wang, and R. National Comorbidity Survey, The epidemiology of major depressive disorder: results from the National Comorbidity Survey Replication (NCS-R). *JAMA,* 2003. 289(23): p. 3095-105.

[168] Washburn, J.J., A.E. West, and J.A. Heil, Treatment of Pediatric Bipolar Disorder: A Review. Minerva Psichiatr, 2011. 52(1): p. 21-35.

[169] Van Meter, A.R., A.L. Moreira, and E.A. Youngstrom, Meta-analysis of epidemiologic studies of pediatric bipolar disorder. *J Clin Psychiatry*, 2011. 72(9): p. 1250-6.

[170] Rajkowska, G., Postmortem studies in mood disorders indicate altered numbers of neurons and glial cells. *Biol Psychiatry*, 2000. 48(8): p. 766-77.

[171] Cotter, D., D. Mackay, S. Landau, R. Kerwin, and I. Everall, Reduced glial cell density and neuronal size in the anterior cingulate cortex in major depressive disorder. *Arch Gen Psychiatry*, 2001. 58(6): p. 545-53.

[172] Sacher, J., J. Neumann, T. Funfstuck, A. Soliman, A. Villringer, and M.L. Schroeter, Mapping the depressed brain: a meta-analysis of structural and functional alterations in major depressive disorder. *J Affect Disord*, 2012. 140(2): p. 142-8.

[173] Femenia, T., M. Gomez-Galan, M. Lindskog, and S. Magara, Dysfunctional hippocampal activity affects emotion and cognition in mood disorders. *Brain Res,* 2012. 1476: p. 58-70.

[174] Si, X., J.J. Miguel-Hidalgo, G. O'Dwyer, C.A. Stockmeier, and G. Rajkowska, Age-dependent reductions in the level of glial fibrillary acidic protein in the prefrontal cortex in major depression. *Neuropsychopharmacology,* 2004. 29(11): p. 2088-96.

[175] Torres-Platas, S.G., C. Hercher, M.A. Davoli, G. Maussion, B. Labonte, G. Turecki, and N. Mechawar, Astrocytic hypertrophy in anterior cingulate white matter of depressed suicides. *Neuropsychopharmacology*, 2011. 36(13): p. 2650-8.

[176] Vostrikov, V. and N. Uranova, Age-related increase in the number of oligodendrocytes is dysregulated in schizophrenia and mood disorders. *Schizophr Res Treatment*, 2011. 2011:174689.

[177] Hamidi, M., W.C. Drevets, and J.L. Price, Glial reduction in amygdala in major depressive disorder is due to oligodendrocytes. *Biol Psychiatry*, 2004. 55(6): p. 563-9.

[178] Almeida, J.R., A. Versace, A. Mechelli, S. Hassel, K. Quevedo, D.J. Kupfer, and M.L. Phillips, Abnormal amygdala-prefrontal effective connectivity to happy faces differentiates bipolar from major depression. *Biol Psychiatry,* 2009. 66(5): p. 451-9.

[179] Rothermundt, M., V. Arolt, M. Wiesmann, U. Missler, M. Peters, S. Rudolf, and H. Kirchner, S-100B is increased in melancholic but not in non-melancholic major depression. *J Affect Disord*, 2001. 66(1): p. 89-93.

[180] Schroeter, M.L. and J. Steiner, Elevated serum levels of the glial marker protein S100B are not specific for schizophrenia or mood disorders. *Mol Psychiatry*, 2009. 14(3): p. 235-7.

[181] Schroeter, M.L., J. Steiner, and K. Mueller, Glial pathology is modified by age in mood disorders--a systematic meta-analysis of serum S100B in vivo studies. *J Affect Disord,* 2011. 134(1-3): p. 32-8.

[182] Luo, K.R., C.J. Hong, Y.J. Liou, S.J. Hou, Y.H. Huang, and S.J. Tsai, Differential regulation of neurotrophin S100B and BDNF in two rat models of depression. *Prog Neuropsychopharmacol Biol Psychiatry,* 2010. 34(8): p. 1433-9.

[183] Schroeter, M.L., H. Abdul-Khaliq, M. Krebs, A. Diefenbacher, and I.E. Blasig, Serum markers support disease-specific glial pathology in major depression. *J Affect Disord*, 2008. 111(2-3): p. 271-80.

[184] Grabe, H.J., N. Ahrens, H.J. Rose, C. Kessler, and H.J. Freyberger, Neurotrophic factor S100 beta in major depression. *Neuropsychobiology,* 2001. 44(2): p. 88-90.

[185] Machado-Vieira, R., A.P. Schmidt, T.T. Avila, F. Kapczinski, J.C. Soares, D.O. Souza, and L.V. Portela, Increased cerebrospinal fluid levels of S100B protein in rat model of mania induced by ouabain. *Life Sci,* 2004. 76(7): p. 805-11.

[186] Dean, B., L. Gray, and E. Scarr, Regionally specific changes in levels of cortical S100beta in bipolar 1 disorder but not schizophrenia. *Aust N Z J Psychiatry,* 2006. 40(3): p. 217-24.

[187] Rong, H., G. Wang, T. Liu, H. Wang, Q. Wan, and S. Weng, Chronic mild stress induces fluoxetine-reversible decreases in hippocampal and cerebrospinal fluid levels of the neurotrophic factor S100B and its specific receptor. *Int J Mol Sci,* 2010. 11(12): p. 5310-22.

[188] Gos, T., M.L. Schroeter, W. Lessel, H.G. Bernstein, H. Dobrowolny, K. Schiltz, B. Bogerts, and J. Steiner, S100B-immunopositive astrocytes and oligodendrocytes in the hippocampus are differentially afflicted in unipolar and bipolar depression: a postmortem study. *J Psychiatr Res,* 2013. 47(11): p. 1694-9.

[189] Kawaguchi, Y., T. Okamoto, M. Taniwaki, M. Aizawa, M. Inoue, S. Katayama, H. Kawakami, S. Nakamura, M. Nishimura, I. Akiguchi, and et al., CAG expansions in a novel gene for Machado-Joseph disease at chromosome 14q32.1. *Nat Genet,* 1994. 8(3): p. 221-8.

[190] Kawakami, H., H. Maruyama, S. Nakamura, Y. Kawaguchi, A. Kakizuka, M. Doyu, and G. Sobue, Unique features of the CAG repeats in Machado-Joseph disease. *Nat Genet,* 1995. 9(4): p. 344-5.

[191] Seidel, K., S. Siswanto, E.R. Brunt, W. den Dunnen, H.W. Korf, and U. Rub, Brain pathology of spinocerebellar ataxias. *Acta Neuropathol,* 2012. 124(1): p. 1-21.

[192] C. Franca M, J., A. D'Abreu, A. Nucci, F. Cendes, and I. Lopes-Cendes, Prospective study of peripheral neuropathy in Machado-Joseph disease. *Muscle Nerve*, 2009. 40(6): p. 1012-8.

[193] Klockgether, T., L. Schols, M. Abele, K. Burk, H. Topka, F. Andres, G. Amoiridis, R. Ludtke, O. Riess, F. Laccone, and J. Dichgans, Age related axonal neuropathy in spinocerebellar ataxia type 3/Machado-Joseph disease (SCA3/MJD). *J Neurol Neurosurg Psychiatry*, 1999. 66(2): p. 222-4.

[194] Suga, N., M. Katsuno, H. Koike, H. Banno, K. Suzuki, A. Hashizume, T. Mano, M. Iijima, Y. Kawagashira, M. Hirayama, T. Nakamura, H. Watanabe, F. Tanaka, and G. Sobue, Schwann cell involvement in the peripheral neuropathy of spinocerebellar ataxia type 3. *Neuropathol Appl Neurobiol*, 2014. 40(5): p. 628-39.

[195] Tort, A.B., L.V. Portela, I.C. Rockenbach, T.L. Monte, M.L. Pereira, D.O. Souza, C.R. Rieder, and L.B. Jardim, S100B and NSE serum concentrations in Machado Joseph disease. *Clin Chim Acta*, 2005. 351(1-2): p. 143-8.

[196] Zhou, J., L. Lei, Y. Shi, J. Wang, H. Jiang, L. Shen, and B. Tang, Serum concentrations of NSE and S100B in spinocerebellar ataxia type 3/Machado-Joseph disease. *Zhong Nan Da Xue Xue Bao Yi Xue Ban,* 2011. 36(6): p. 504-10.

[197] Vucic, S., M.C. Kiernan, and D.R. Cornblath, Guillain-Barre syndrome: an update. *J Clin Neurosci,* 2009. 16(6): p. 733-41.

[198] Sharshar, T., S. Chevret, F. Bourdain, J.C. Raphael, and S. French Cooperative Group on Plasma Exchange in Guillain-Barre, Early predictors of mechanical ventilation in Guillain-Barre syndrome. *Crit Care Med*, 2003. 31(1): p. 278-83.

[199] Dornonville de la Cour, C., H. Andersen, E. Stalberg, A. Fuglsang-Frederiksen, and J. Jakobsen, Electrophysiological signs of permanent axonal loss in a follow-up study of patients with Guillain-Barre syndrome. *Muscle Nerve*, 2005. 31(1): p. 70-7.

[200] Prineas, J.W., Pathology of the Guillain-Barre syndrome. *Ann Neurol,* 1981. 9 Suppl: p. 6-19.

[201] Hafer-Macko, C., S.T. Hsieh, C.Y. Li, T.W. Ho, K. Sheikh, D.R. Cornblath, G.M. McKhann, A.K. Asbury, and J.W. Griffin, Acute motor axonal neuropathy: an antibody-mediated attack on axolemma. *Ann Neurol,* 1996. 40(4): p. 635-44.

[202] Mokuno, K., K. Kiyosawa, K. Sugimura, T. Yasuda, S. Riku, T. Murayama, T. Yanagi, A. Takahashi, and K. Kato, Prognostic value of

cerebrospinal fluid neuron-specific enolase and S-100b protein in Guillain-Barre syndrome. *Acta Neurol Scand*, 1994. 89(1): p. 27-30.
[203] Petzold, A., J. Brettschneider, K. Jin, G. Keir, N.M. Murray, N.P. Hirsch, Y. Itoyama, M.M. Reilly, A. Takeda, and H. Tumani, CSF protein biomarkers for proximal axonal damage improve prognostic accuracy in the acute phase of Guillain-Barre syndrome. *Muscle Nerve*, 2009. 40(1): p. 42-9.
[204] Wang, X.K., H.L. Zhang, F.H. Meng, M. Chang, Y.Z. Wang, T. Jin, E. Mix, and J. Zhu, Elevated levels of S100B, tau and pNFH in cerebrospinal fluid are correlated with subtypes of Guillain-Barre syndrome. *Neurol Sci,* 2013. 34(5): p. 655-61.
[205] Piazza, O., G. Esposito, E. De Robertis, G. Servillo, and R. Tufano, S100B in Guillain-Barre syndrome. *Br J Anaesth*, 2006. 96(1): p. 141-2.
[206] Trapp, B.D. and K.A. Nave, Multiple sclerosis: an immune or neurodegenerative disorder? Annu Rev Neurosci, 2008. 31: p. 247-69.
[207] Koch-Henriksen, N. and P.S. Sorensen, The changing demographic pattern of multiple sclerosis epidemiology. *Lancet Neurol*, 2010. 9(5): p. 520-32.
[208] Baranzini, S.E., The genetics of autoimmune diseases: a networked perspective. *Curr Opin Immunol*, 2009. 21(6): p. 596-605.
[209] Baranzini, S.E., J. Wang, R.A. Gibson, N. Galwey, Y. Naegelin, F. Barkhof, E.W. Radue, R.L. Lindberg, B.M. Uitdehaag, M.R. Johnson, A. Angelakopoulou, L. Hall, J.C. Richardson, R.K. Prinjha, A. Gass, J.J. Geurts, J. Kragt, M. Sombekke, H. Vrenken, P. Qualley, R.R. Lincoln, R. Gomez, S.J. Caillier, M.F. George, H. Mousavi, R. Guerrero, D.T. Okuda, B.A. Cree, A.J. Green, E. Waubant, D.S. Goodin, D. Pelletier, P.M. Matthews, S.L. Hauser, L. Kappos, C.H. Polman, and J.R. Oksenberg, Genome-wide association analysis of susceptibility and clinical phenotype in multiple sclerosis. *Hum Mol Genet*, 2009. 18(4): p. 767-78.
[210] Chard, D. and D. Miller, Is multiple sclerosis a generalized disease of the central nervous system? An MRI perspective. *Curr Opin Neurol,* 2009. 22(3): p. 214-8.
[211] Ferguson, B., M.K. Matyszak, M.M. Esiri, and V.H. Perry, Axonal damage in acute multiple sclerosis lesions. *Brain,* 1997. 120 (Pt 3): p. 393-9.
[212] Kuhlmann, T., G. Lingfeld, A. Bitsch, J. Schuchardt, and W. Bruck, Acute axonal damage in multiple sclerosis is most extensive in early

disease stages and decreases over time. *Brain,* 2002. 125(Pt 10): p. 2202-12.

[213] Trapp, B.D., J. Peterson, R.M. Ransohoff, R. Rudick, S. Mork, and L. Bo, Axonal transection in the lesions of multiple sclerosis. *N Engl J Med,* 1998. 338(5): p. 278-85.

[214] Smith, K.J. and H. Lassmann, The role of nitric oxide in multiple sclerosis. *Lancet Neurol,* 2002. 1(4): p. 232-41.

[215] Massaro, A.R., F. Michetti, A. Laudisio, and P. Bergonzi, Myelin basic protein and S-100 antigen in cerebrospinal fluid of patients with multiple sclerosis in the acute phase. *Ital J Neurol Sci*, 1985. 6(1): p. 53-6.

[216] Lamers, K.J., B.G. van Engelen, F.J. Gabreels, O.R. Hommes, G.F. Borm, and R.A. Wevers, Cerebrospinal neuron-specific enolase, S-100 and myelin basic protein in neurological disorders. *Acta Neurol Scand,* 1995. 92(3): p. 247-51.

[217] Bartosik-Psujek, H., M. Psujek, J. Jaworski, and Z. Stelmasiak, Total tau and S100b proteins in different types of multiple sclerosis and during immunosuppressive treatment with mitoxantrone. *Acta Neurol Scand,* 2011. 123(4): p. 252-6.

[218] Missler, U., K.P. Wandinger, M. Wiesmann, M. Kaps, and K. Wessel, Acute exacerbation of multiple sclerosis increases plasma levels of S-100 protein. *Acta Neurol Scand*, 1997. 96(3): p. 142-4.

[219] Markowitz, J., A.D. MacKerell, Jr., and D.J. Weber, A search for inhibitors of S100B, a member of the S100 family of calcium-binding proteins. *Mini Rev Med Chem*, 2007. 7(6): p. 609-16.

[220] Donato, R., Chlorpromazine inhibits the calcium-mediated effects of S-100 protein(s) on assembled brain microtubule proteins, but not those on microtubule protein assembly. *Biochem Biophys Res Commun*, 1984. 122(3): p. 983-90.

[221] Smith, J., B.J. Stewart, S. Glaysher, K. Peregrin, L.A. Knight, D.J. Weber, and I.A. Cree, The effect of pentamidine on melanoma ex vivo. *Anticancer Drugs*, 2010. 21(2): p. 181-5.

[222] Esposito, G., E. Capoccia, G. Sarnelli, C. Scuderi, C. Cirillo, R. Cuomo, and L. Steardo, The antiprotozoal drug pentamidine ameliorates experimentally induced acute colitis in mice. *J Neuroinflammation*, 2012. 9:277.

[223] Van Wauwe, J., F. Aerts, H. Van Genechten, H. Blockx, W. Deleersnijder, and H. Walter, The inhibitory effect of pentamidine on the production of chemotactic cytokines by in vitro stimulated human blood cells. *Inflamm Res*, 1996. 45(7): p. 357-63.

[224] Rosenthal, G.J., E. Corsini, W.A. Craig, C.E. Comment, and M.I. Luster, Pentamidine: an inhibitor of interleukin-1 that acts via a post-translational event. *Toxicol Appl Pharmacol*, 1991. 107(3): p. 555-61.

[225] Corsini, E., W.A. Craig, and G.J. Rosenthal, Modulation of tumor necrosis factor release from alveolar macrophages treated with pentamidine isethionate. *Int J Immunopharmacol*, 1992. 14(2): p. 121-30.

[226] Cirillo, C., E. Capoccia, T. Iuvone, R. Cuomo, G. Sarnelli, L. Steardo, and G. Esposito, S100B Inhibitor Pentamidine Attenuates Reactive Gliosis and Reduces Neuronal Loss in a Mouse Model of Alzheimer's Disease. *BioMed Research International*, 2014. 508342.

[227] Vig, P.J., S. Hearst, Q. Shao, M.E. Lopez, H.A. Murphy, 2nd, and E. Safaya, Glial S100B protein modulates mutant ataxin-1 aggregation and toxicity: TRTK12 peptide, a potential candidate for SCA1 therapy. *Cerebellum,* 2011. 10(2): p. 254-66.

[228] Deane, R., I. Singh, A.P. Sagare, R.D. Bell, N.T. Ross, B. LaRue, R. Love, S. Perry, N. Paquette, R.J. Deane, M. Thiyagarajan, T. Zarcone, G. Fritz, A.E. Friedman, B.L. Miller, and B.V. Zlokovic, A multimodal RAGE-specific inhibitor reduces amyloid beta-mediated brain disorder in a mouse model of Alzheimer disease. *J Clin Invest*, 2012. 122(4): p. 1377-92.

[229] Pan, W., P. Xin, S. Patrick, S. Dean, C. Keating, and G. Clawson, Primer-free aptamer selection using a random DNA library. *J Vis Exp,* 2010. 41:2039.

[230] Rohde, D., J. Ritterhoff, M. Voelkers, H.A. Katus, T.G. Parker, and P. Most, S100A1: a multifaceted therapeutic target in cardiovascular disease. *J Cardiovasc Transl Res*, 2010. 3(5): p. 525-37.

[231] van Dieck, J., D.P. Teufel, A.M. Jaulent, M.R. Fernandez-Fernandez, T.J. Rutherford, A. Wyslouch-Cieszynska, and A.R. Fersht, Posttranslational modifications affect the interaction of S100 proteins with tumor suppressor p53. *J Mol Biol*, 2009. 394(5): p. 922-30.

[232] Kizawa, K., H. Takahara, M. Unno, and C.W. Heizmann, S100 and S100 fused-type protein families in epidermal maturation with special focus on S100A3 in mammalian hair cuticles. *Biochimie,* 2011. 93(12): p. 2038-47.

[233] Stein, U., F. Arlt, W. Walther, J. Smith, T. Waldman, E.D. Harris, S.D. Mertins, C.W. Heizmann, D. Allard, W. Birchmeier, P.M. Schlag, and R.H. Shoemaker, The metastasis-associated gene S100A4 is a novel

target of beta-catenin/T-cell factor signaling in colon cancer. *Gastroenterology,* 2006. 131(5): p. 1486-500.

[234] Glaser, R., J. Harder, H. Lange, J. Bartels, E. Christophers, and J.M. Schroder, Antimicrobial psoriasin (S100A7) protects human skin from Escherichia coli infection. *Nat Immunol*, 2005. 6(1): p. 57-64.

[235] Sinha, P., C. Okoro, D. Foell, H.H. Freeze, S. Ostrand-Rosenberg, and G. Srikrishna, Proinflammatory S100 proteins regulate the accumulation of myeloid-derived suppressor cells. *J Immunol*, 2008. 181(7): p. 4666-75.

[236] Ikemoto, M., H. Murayama, H. Itoh, M. Totani, and M. Fujita, Intrinsic function of S100A8/A9 complex as an anti-inflammatory protein in liver injury induced by lipopolysaccharide in rats. *Clin Chim Acta*, 2007. 376(1-2): p. 197-204.

[237] Yang, X., N.C. Popescu, and D.B. Zimonjic, DLC1 interaction with S100A10 mediates inhibition of in vitro cell invasion and tumorigenicity of lung cancer cells through a RhoGAP-independent mechanism. *Cancer Res,* 2011. 71(8): p. 2916-25.

[238] O'Connell, P.A., A.P. Surette, R.S. Liwski, P. Svenningsson, and D.M. Waisman, S100A10 regulates plasminogen-dependent macrophage invasion. *Blood*, 2010. 116(7): p. 1136-46.

[239] Sakaguchi, M., H. Sonegawa, H. Murata, M. Kitazoe, J. Futami, K. Kataoka, H. Yamada, and N.H. Huh, S100A11, an dual mediator for growth regulation of human keratinocytes. *Mol Biol Cell*, 2008. 19(1): p. 78-85.

[240] Yang, Z., W.X. Yan, H. Cai, N. Tedla, C. Armishaw, N. Di Girolamo, H.W. Wang, T. Hampartzoumian, J.L. Simpson, P.G. Gibson, J. Hunt, P. Hart, J.M. Hughes, M.A. Perry, P.F. Alewood, and C.L. Geczy, S100A12 provokes mast cell activation: a potential amplification pathway in asthma and innate immunity. *J Allergy Clin Immunol*, 2007. 119(1): p. 106-14.

[241] Mikkelsen, S.E., V. Novitskaya, M. Kriajevska, V. Berezin, E. Bock, B. Norrild, and E. Lukanidin, S100A12 protein is a strong inducer of neurite outgrowth from primary hippocampal neurons. *J Neurochem,* 2001. 79(4): p. 767-76.

[242] Hsieh, H.L., B.W. Schafer, B. Weigle, and C.W. Heizmann, S100 protein translocation in response to extracellular S100 is mediated by receptor for advanced glycation endproducts in human endothelial cells. *Biochem Biophys Res Commun*, 2004. 316(3): p. 949-59.

[243] Kathir, K.M., K. Ibrahim, D. Rajalingam, I. Prudovsky, C. Yu, and T.K. Kumar, S100A13-lipid interactions-role in the non-classical release of the acidic fibroblast growth factor. *Biochim Biophys Acta*, 2007. 1768(12): p. 3080-9.

[244] Chen, H., Y. Yuan, C. Zhang, A. Luo, F. Ding, J. Ma, S. Yang, Y. Tian, T. Tong, Q. Zhan, and Z. Liu, Involvement of S100A14 protein in cell invasion by affecting expression and function of matrix metalloproteinase (MMP)-2 via p53-dependent transcriptional regulation. *J Biol Chem,* 2012. 287(21): p. 17109-19.

[245] Liu, Y., R. Zhang, J. Xin, Y. Sun, J. Li, D. Wei, and A.Z. Zhao, Identification of S100A16 as a novel adipogenesis promoting factor in 3T3-L1 cells. *Endocrinology*, 2011. 152(3): p. 903-11.

[246] Malmendal, A., C.W. Vander Kooi, N.C. Nielsen, and W.J. Chazin, Calcium-modulated S100 protein-phospholipid interactions. An NMR study of calbindin D9k and DPC. *Biochemistry,* 2005. 44(17): p. 6502-12.

[247] Arumugam, T. and C.D. Logsdon, S100P: a novel therapeutic target for cancer. *Amino Acids*, 2011. 41(4): p. 893-9.

[248] Lee, S.C., I.G. Kim, L.N. Marekov, E.J. O'Keefe, D.A. Parry, and P.M. Steinert, The structure of human trichohyalin. Potential multiple roles as a functional EF-hand-like calcium-binding protein, a cornified cell envelope precursor, and an intermediate filament-associated (cross-linking) protein. *J Biol Chem*, 1993. 268(16): p. 12164-76.

[249] Portela, L.C., A.B. Tort, E.C. Neto, R.G. Kessler, V. Penchaszadeh, D.O. Souza, C.A. Goncalves, and R. Giugliani, High immunocontent of S100 beta protein in amniotic fluid of pregnancies with Down syndrome. *Ultrasound Obstet Gynecol*, 2000. 16(6): p. 590-2.

[250] Gazzolo, D., M. Bruschettini, V. Corvino, M. Lituania, R. Sarli, P. Bruschettini, and F. Michetti, Amniotic fluid levels of S100B protein in normal and trisomy-21 foetuses. *Clin Chim Acta*, 2003. 330(1-2): p. 131-3.

[251] Mito, T. and L.E. Becker, Developmental changes of S-100 protein and glial fibrillary acidic protein in the brain in Down syndrome. *Exp Neurol,* 1993. 120(2): p. 170-6.

[252] Lara, D.R., C.S. Gama, P. Belmonte-de-Abreu, L.V. Portela, C.A. Goncalves, M. Fonseca, S. Hauck, and D.O. Souza, Increased serum S100B protein in schizophrenia: a study in medication-free patients. *J Psychiatr Res,* 2001. 35(1): p. 11-4.

[253] Schmitt, A., T. Bertsch, U. Henning, H. Tost, A. Klimke, F.A. Henn, and P. Falkai, Increased serum S100B in elderly, chronic schizophrenic patients: negative correlation with deficit symptoms. *Schizophr Res,* 2005. 80(2-3): p. 305-13.

[254] Schroeter, M.L., H. Abdul-Khaliq, M. Krebs, A. Diefenbacher, and I.E. Blasig, Neuron-specific enolase is unaltered whereas S100B is elevated in serum of patients with schizophrenia--original research and meta-analysis. *Psychiatry Res,* 2009. 167(1-2): p. 66-72.

[255] Zhang, X.Y., M.H. Xiu, C. Chen da, F.Y. Zhu, G.Y. Wu, C.N. Haile, L. Lu, T.A. Kosten, and T.R. Kosten, Increased S100B serum levels in schizophrenic patients with tardive dyskinesia: association with dyskinetic movements. *J Psychiatr Res*, 2010. 44(7): p. 429-33.

[256] Hof, P.R., V. Haroutunian, V.L. Friedrich, Jr., W. Byne, C. Buitron, D.P. Perl, and K.L. Davis, Loss and altered spatial distribution of oligodendrocytes in the superior frontal gyrus in schizophrenia. *Biol Psychiatry,* 2003. 53(12): p. 1075-85.

[257] Stark, A.K., H.B. Uylings, E. Sanz-Arigita, and B. Pakkenberg, Glial cell loss in the anterior cingulate cortex, a subregion of the prefrontal cortex, in subjects with schizophrenia. *Am J Psychiatry,* 2004. 161(5): p. 882-8.

[258] Byne, W., S. Dracheva, B. Chin, J.M. Schmeidler, K.L. Davis, and V. Haroutunian, Schizophrenia and sex associated differences in the expression of neuronal and oligodendrocyte-specific genes in individual thalamic nuclei. *Schizophr Res*, 2008. 98(1-3): p. 118-28.

[259] Tkachev, D., M.L. Mimmack, M.M. Ryan, M. Wayland, T. Freeman, P.B. Jones, M. Starkey, M.J. Webster, R.H. Yolken, and S. Bahn, Oligodendrocyte dysfunction in schizophrenia and bipolar disorder. *Lancet,* 2003. 362(9386): p. 798-805.

[260] Kanaan, R.A., J.S. Kim, W.E. Kaufmann, G.D. Pearlson, G.J. Barker, and P.K. McGuire, Diffusion tensor imaging in schizophrenia. *Biol Psychiatry,* 2005. 58(12): p. 921-9.

[261] Kubicki, M., R.W. McCarley, and M.E. Shenton, Evidence for white matter abnormalities in schizophrenia. *Curr Opin Psychiatry*, 2005. 18(2): p. 121-34.

[262] Hayashi, Y., N. Nihonmatsu-Kikuchi, X. Yu, K. Ishimoto, S.I. Hisanaga, and Y. Tatebayashi, A novel, rapid, quantitative cell-counting method reveals oligodendroglial reduction in the frontopolar cortex in major depressive disorder. *Mol Psychiatry*, 2011. 16(12): p. 1155-8.
[263] Hughes, R.A. and D.R. Cornblath, Guillain-Barre syndrome. *Lancet,* 2005. 366(9497): p. 1653-66.

Index

A

B

C

D

E

F

G

H

I

K

L

M

N

O

P

Q

R

S

T

U

V

W

Y

Z